The International Librar
T0229966

A NEGLECTED COMPLEX AND ITS RELATION TO FREUDIAN PSYCHOLOGY

ARBOR SCIENTIÆ
ARBOR VITÆ

Founded by C. K. Ogden

The International Library of Psychology

PSYCHOANALYSIS
In 28 Volumes

I	The Elements of Practical Psycho-Analysis	*Bousfield*
II	A Neglected Complex and its Relation to Freudian Psychology	*Bousfield*
III	The Omnipotent Self	*Bousfield*
IV	The Social Basis of Consciousness	*Burrow*
V	What is Psychoanalysis?	*Coriat*
VI	The Psychoanalytic Theory of Neurosis	*Fenichel*
VII	The Technique of Psycho-Analysis	*Forsyth*
VIII	Leonardo da Vinci	*Freud*
IX	Totem and Taboo	*Freud*
X	Wit and its Relation to the Unconscious	*Freud*
XI	Morbid Fears and Compulsions	*Frink*
XII	Facts and Theories of Psychoanalysis	*Hendrick*
XIII	Fathers or Sons?	*Hopkins*
XIV	Neurosis and Human Growth	*Horney*
XV	The Neurotic Personality of Our Time	*Horney*
XVI	New Ways in Psychoanalysis	*Horney*
XVII	Our Inner Conflicts	*Horney*
XVIII	Self-Analysis	*Horney*
XIX	Childhood and After	*Isaacs*
XX	Social Development in Young Children	*Isaacs*
XXI	Problems in Psychopathology	*Mitchell*
XXII	The Psychoanalytic Method	*Pfister*
XXIII	The Trauma of Birth	*Rank*
XXIV	On the Bringing Up of Children	*Rickman*
XXV	Conflict and Dream	*Rivers*
XXVI	Psychoanalysis and Suggestion Therapy	*Stekel*
XXVII	Psychoanalysis and Behaviour	*Tridon*
XXVIII	Character and the Unconscious	*van der Hoop*

A NEGLECTED COMPLEX AND ITS RELATION TO FREUDIAN PSYCHOLOGY

W R BOUSFIELD

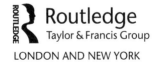

Routledge
Taylor & Francis Group
LONDON AND NEW YORK

First published in 1924 by
Routledge, Trench, Trubner & Co., Ltd.
2 Park Square, Milton Park, Abingdon, Oxfordshire OX14 4RN
711 Third Avenue, New York, NY 10017

First issued in paperback 2014

Routledge is an imprint of the Taylor and Francis Group, an informa business

British Library Cataloguing in Publication Data
A CIP catalogue record for this book
is available from the British Library

A Neglected Complex and its Relation to Freudian Psychology
ISBN 0415-21083-6
Psychoanalysis: 28 Volumes
ISBN 0415-21132-8
The International Library of Psychology: 204 Volumes
ISBN 0415-19132-7

ISBN 13: 978-1-138-87553-1 (pbk)
ISBN 13: 978-0-415-21083-6 (hbk)

PREFACE

SOME of the ideas which are elaborated in this book have been already foreshadowed in two papers by the author on *Telepathy* (Hibbert Journal, April 1922) and *Human Survival* (Hibbert Journal, April 1924). Also in a paper on *Determinism in relation to Psycho-analysis* (*Psyche, No. 2*) by the author and Dr. Paul Bousfield, and in the *Elements of Practical Psycho-analysis* by the latter; to whom the author is indebted for reading the proofs and valuable suggestions. To show the effect of these ideas in modifying the Freudian psychology is the purpose of this book.

W.R.B.

St. Swithin's, Northwood.
15th July, 1924.

CONTENTS

Chapter.   Page.

  I. INTRODUCTION   ··   ··   ··   ··   1

 II. SOME FEATURES OF FREUD'S PSYCHOLOGY   12

III. THE MATERIALISTIC COMPLEX   ··   ··   18

 IV. FREE-WILL AND DETERMINISM   ··   ··   39

  V. TOTEM AND TABOO   ··   ··   ··   48

 VI. LOVE, 'Αγάπη AMOR   ··   ··   ··   61

VII. ENERGY   ··   ··   ··   ··   ··   68

VIII. WILL POWER   ··   ··   ··   ··   82

 IX. THE WILL AS A DETERMINANT   ··   ··   92

  X. SUGGESTION   ··   ··   ··   ··   100

 XI. CONCLUSIONS   ··   ··   ··   ··   111

A Neglected Complex

CHAPTER I

INTRODUCTION

THE work of Freud in unravelling the mysteries of the unconscious mind is a psychological achievement of the highest import. Thanks to him we know that many of our most important mental activities proceed entirely outside our consciousness in the hidden caverns of the mind. These dark caves of the unconscious are revealed to us not merely as store-houses but as power-houses, where the springs of action are hidden from ourselves. We have learned that a large part of our active life is motivated from this unconscious power-house.

Day by day in life there occur in our consciousness conflicts between duty and inclination, between the thoughts of pleasure and of the consequences which may ensue, in fact any kind of pull between opposing motives for and against any given action. All these conflicts leave their hidden traces in the unconscious mind

and there become involved in a mental mechanism on which Freud has thrown the searchlight
of analysis. All this and more is of great value
and capable of being used in ways which Freud
has not explored.

Were it not for the high value of the structure
of knowledge which Freud has built, it would
not be worth while to seek for and examine the
defects in the building. The valuable part of
Freud's discoveries is independent of and
separable from the rest. The ore which he has
worked is rich, but the baser metal must be
eliminated if the fine gold is to be utilized.

It may be said at once that the chief defects
of Freud's psychology arise from a complex of
which he is unconscious and which leads him to
interpret all psychic phenomena in terms of
materialism. The notions of God, of human
survival and of free-will are for him myths or
illusions. Mind is a function of the material
brain and perishes with it. These things he
holds not merely as philosophic speculations,
but he has attempted to prove them by a
specious psychological camouflage which we
shall examine in due course. The age-long
distinction between the σῶμα which perishes
and the ψυχή which survives, going back far
beyond the Greeks to the most primitive races,
and still for mankind at large a vital belief, is

for him non-existent. The distinction is of importance not only for a sound psychology but also for psycho-therapy. A psychology which fails in its appreciation of the highest qualities of the psyche, and recognizes only those attributes which spring from the constitution of the soma, should rather be called somatology than psychology. Thus, for instance, love in its highest form—the love which " seeketh not its own " and whose end is giving rather than getting—is an attribute of the psyche and not of the soma. But, according to Freud, it is a sort of sublimation or diversion of sexual impulses. So also is the psychic energy which has led the pioneers of the human race to the achievement of great and noble' ends in the service of mankind. This love and this energy are psychological facts which are not to be degraded from their true place by analogies drawn from analytical researches made upon abnormal patients who are the very last persons we should take as representatives of human nature at its best.

But this confusion of the psyche and the soma is as destructive for psycho-therapy as it is for pure psychological science. With an engineer or even a surgeon materialism would not necessarily affect his professional work. But in the realm of psycho-therapy it cannot but make much difference, whether the physician works on the hypothesis that the pysche has or has not a real existence independent of the body. If the psyche survives then the character of the surviving personality is of the highest importance ; for character, in its broad sense, including the capacities and the springs which regulate thought and action, will be the one and only thing which the psyche carries over into the next life, and is therefore the thing that is of permanent value. If the psyche does not survive then health and happiness for the remaining years of the patient's life are all that the physician need envisage. What matter if these can be gained at the expense of character ! No one would suggest that the materialist physician would unnecessarily sacrifice character, but if it came to the question of saving the mother or the child, he would unhesitatingly sacrifice the child—*character*. That Freud's materialism does enter into his therapy no one who reads his lectures can deny. But it is possible to get all the therapeutic advantage of Freud's discoveries without incurring the consequences of his materialism. To help separate the chaff from the wheat is the main object of these criticisms. It is for the practitioner to utilize the wheat. Our chief object is to show that some of the chaff may be eliminated, and that without the chaff Freud's discoveries may lead to greater and more useful results.

It is strange that Freud's psychology should lead him to materialism, for it contains principles which should have warned him against this development. It will be shown that he suffers from a materialistic complex which disables him from useful thought in the realm of speculative philosophy. This complex is generated and gives rise to " compulsion ideas " in the precise way which he has expounded in reference to those complexes which are the subject of his discoveries. This neglected complex is entirely unknown to him, and, on the principles which we owe to his analytic genius, it cannot be discovered by self-analysis, nor by the analysis of his strict followers who are afflicted with the same complex. He suffers from it in common with some physical scientists who, unknown to themselves, also display the symptoms which arise from the materialistic complex. The unfortunate thing about it is that, not only is the force and operation of this complex entirely unknown to the sufferers, but that there is no real chance of bringing it to light so that they may become conscious of it. They suffer from it and in the absence of some unlikely mental upheaval they must continue to suffer from it.

These criticisms will therefore be of no use to them, but it is hoped that they may be useful to those in whom the complex is not fully developed. It is possible that analysis by a therapist who does not suffer from the complex might bring it into consciousness, but the resistances would probably be too great to make the analysis useful, and indeed the materialistic complex, when fully developed, would prevent the patient from submitting himself to such analysis. But for those who are not yet caught in its meshes these criticisms will be useful.

It should be observed that the matters which are involved in the materialistic complex are those matters of belief and opinion in which Freud and his followers, and indeed all psychologists, tell us that a complex is of special potency. Matters of opinion and belief, where no absolute proof is available, are determined by one's mental constellation. Logic is powerless. The content of the unconscious mind determines the opinion.

The questions involved in the doctrines of materialism are incapable of logical proof one way or another, and the scientist who goes out of his way, that is the way of pure science, to preach materialism, is dogmatising about matters of opinion and belief in which his conclusions are determined not by scientific facts but by the content of his unconscious mind, of which in such matters the materialistic complex is the most potent, and of which he is necessarily ignorant. Freud professes to have arrived at his materialism by psychological deductions, but these deductions, being in the realm of opinion, are not the less governed by his materialistic complex because he is a psychologist. When he says[1] :—

" As a matter of fact, I believe that a large part of the mythological conception of the world which reaches far into the most modern religions *is nothing but psychology projected into the outer world.*"

he is expressing a mere opinion which, in accordance with the principles of his psychology, is solely the result of his mental constellation, and has no basis in fact or in logic. And when referring to the analogy of paranoia he continues :

" We venture to explain in this way the myths of paradise and the fall of man, of God, of good and evil, of immortality and the like."

it is his materialistic complex, all unknown to himself, which dictates this analogy and the sweeping and destructive deductions which he

---

[1] Psycho-pathology of Everyday Life p. 309. T. Fisher Unwin Ltd.

bases upon it. And this materialism and its consequences he carries into his psycho-therapy.

We propose to deal somewhat fully with the psychological camouflage by which Freud attempts to support his materialism. Our discussion of the materialistic complex will also throw light on the materialism of some physical scientists. Their attitude becomes less and less excusable as science advances.

Physiology has furnished many materialists who have concluded that mind is a mere function of brain. But the recent work of Dr Head[1] in relation to injuries of the brain which result in aphasia, indicates the reverse conclusion, viz., that the brain is a mere organ of the mind, and that though the brain is injured, the mind may remain intact. He has described cases of aphasia in which, whilst the brain is so injured that it is incapable of initiating spoken words for ideas in the mind, so that some other symbol has to be used for conveying the ideas, *yet the general intelligence is unaffected.* Thus an aphasic may be able to play chess although he cannot name the pieces on the board. The *organ* of the mind is injured, but the mind itself is uninjured. Thus we have noteworthy scientific evidence that although the mind is

---

[1] *Speech and Cerebral Localization,* by Henry Head: *Brain,* vol. xlvi., Part IV. 1923 (Macmillan & Co. Ltd.).

dependent on the brain as its organ for operating on matter, yet the mind itself has existence apart from the material brain, since injuries to the brain do not injure the mind of which the brain is the organ.

Moreover until recent years science rarely looked beyond material phenomena. But matter itself is now shown to be an ethereal phenomenon. We know that the material universe (including our own bodies) is built up of protons and electrons, bathed in and doubtless elaborated from the all-pervading ether. The very simplicity of the basis of the material universe is fatal to the idea that the " fortuitous concourse " of electrons and protons has given birth to all things, including man and his mind.

The mystery of the ether has been so far penetrated that we can conceive of a substance more ethereal than gross matter also elaborated from the ether which, though (like the ether itself), it cannot be detected by our materially-evolved senses, yet may serve as the substratum or vehicle of mind. The immaterial ether has become a concept necessary to our understanding of various phenomena of matter. An ethereal substance which may serve as the vehicle of mind has also become a concept necessary to our comprehension of psychical phenomena.

We know furthermore that the molecules of

which our bodies are composed are aggregations of atoms in which the electrons and protons are spaced so widely apart that the whole body is but an open network in which the constituent protons and electrons occupy but a small fraction of the space which the body appears to occupy. On the hypothesis that the psyche is separated from the soma at death, there is ample room for a psyche interpenetrating the soma composed of ethereal constituents which are no more detectable by our senses than is the ether itself. To postulate the ether in order to account for physical phenomena and to refuse to postulate the ether to account for psychic phenomena is unscientific, and it may be said without fear of contradiction that science reveals nothing which is inconsistent with the separate existence of the psyche and furnishes no grounds for scientific materialism. Indeed the progress of physical science has brought us to a point where it actually suggests that the hypothesis of an ethereal psyche is the only scientific way of accounting for the sporadic yet continually recurring outcrop of psychic phenomena the references to which run all through the course of human history. The hypothesis that all such phenomena are based on illusion is less scientific than the hypothesis of the dual constitution of man—psyche as well as soma, temporarily united, but finally separable—which gives a good account of them.

Further reference will be made to this matter in considering Freud's " Totem and Taboo," in which he endeavours to support his materialistic philosophy by a review of primitive customs and observances on the basis of analogies derived from the mentality of neurotics as disclosed by psycho-analysis. Anyone who is predisposed to materialism by the irksomeness of moral restrictions, is apt to seize upon the doctrines of the professors of materialism, authoritatively propounded by them in the guise of scientific deductions, as affording an easy (but fatal) solution of the moral conflict. For this reason, too, it is important to show that the psychology of Freud and his pupils furnishes no real basis for materialism, which is in fact an illusion which results from a complex of which they are unaware and of which their own psychology rightly applied, furnishes a clear explanation. All that is valuable in Freud's psychology can be utilised without the baneful effects which the materialistic hypothesis brings in its train.

CHAPTER II

ACCORDING to Freud's theory the foundation of a neurosis is to be sought in the unconscious mind.[1] Symptoms are not produced by conscious processes. Every time we meet with a symptom we may conclude that definite unconscious activities which contain the meaning of the symptom are present in the patient's mind.

A symptom shows that some mental process has not been carried through to an end in a normal manner so that it could become conscious. The symptom is a substitute for that which has been repressed. Repression is the essential preliminary condition for the development of symptoms.[2]

To illustrate the relation between the conscious and the unconscious mind Freud[3] compares the unconscious system " to a large ante-room in which the various mental excitations are crowding one upon another like

[1] *Introductory Lectures on Psycho-Analysis*, p. 236. (Geo. Allen & Unwin, Ltd.)
[2] *Loc. cit.* p. 248.   [3] *Loc. cit.* p. 249.

12

individual beings. Adjoining this is a second smaller apartment, a sort of reception room, in which, consciousness resides. But on the threshold of the two there stands a personage with the office of doorkeeper, who examines the various mental excitations, censors them, and denies them admittance to the reception room when he disapproves of them. The excitations in the unconscious, in the ante-chamber, are not visible to consciousness, which is, of course, in the other room, so to begin with they remain unconscious. When they have pressed forward to the threshold and been turned back by the doorkeeper, they are ' incapable of becoming conscious ' ; we call them then repressed."

The motive of the doorkeeper or censor appears to be to keep back excitations of consciousness which would be painful or unpleasant. In Freud's view " Our entire psychical activity is bent upon procuring pleasure and avoiding pain." (p. 298). It is " automatically regulated by the *Pleasure-Principle*."

Freud gives in detail two examples of neuroses (p. 251), and observes : ' What we found in these two examples we should find in every case we submitted to analysis. Every time we should be led by analysis to the sexual desires and experiences of the patient, and every time we should have to affirm that the symptom served the same purpose. This purpose shows itself to be the gratification of sexual wishes—they are a substitute for satisfactions which he does not obtain in reality."

Freud uses the term "libido" to denote the instinctive forces of the sexual life (p. 345). When the libido is turned off or blocked as it were, it must seek an escape by which it can find an outlet for its "charge of energy" (p. 301). Resistance to neurotic illness depends upon the amount of undischarged libido that a person can hold freely suspended and upon how large a portion of it he can deflect from a sexual to a non-sexual goal in sublimation (p. 323). "The fund of energy supporting the symptoms of a neurosis, in every case and regardless of the circumstances inducing their outbreak, is provided by the libido, which is thus put to an abnormal use."

According to Freud (p. 363) the therapeutic effect of psycho-analysis consists in laying bare to the patient the unconscious. By extending the unconscious into consciousness the repressions are raised, the conditions of symptom formation are abolished, and the pathogenic conflict exchanged for a normal one which must be decided one way or the other. Nothing is done for the patients except to enable this one mental change to take place in them.

It is a mistake, he says (p. 362), to imagine that advice and guidance concerning conduct in life forms an integral part of the analytic method. The analyst refrains from playing the part of mentor. He wants the patient to " find his own solutions for himself." Further he observes : " You must not be led away by my eagerness to defend myself against the accusation that in analytic treatment neurotics are encouraged to ' live a free life,' and conclude from it that we influence them in favour of conventional morality. That is at least as far removed from our purpose as the other. We are not reformers, it is true ; we are merely observers ; but we cannot help observing with critical eyes, and we have found it impossible to give our support to conventional sexual morality or to approve of the means by which society attempts to arrange the practical problems of sexuality in life. We can demonstrate with ease that what the world calls its code of morals, demands more sacrifices than it is worth, and that its behaviour is neither dictated by honesty nor instituted with wisdom. We do not absolve our patients from listening to these criticisms, we accustom them to an unprejudiced consideration of sexual matters, like all other matters, and if after they have become independent by the effect of the treatment they choose some intermediate course between unrestrained sexual licence and unconditional asceticism, our conscience is not burdened whatever the outcome."

As a commentary on this may be cited another passage (p. 320) : " To take the commonest case of this kind ; a woman who is brutally treated and mercilessly exploited by her husband fairly regularly takes refuge in a neurosis if her disposition admits of it. This will happen if she is too cowardly or too conventional to console herself secretly with another man.

We reserve our criticisms of the above for later chapters. The kind of " morality " which is exhibited in these quotations is what one might expect from a psychology which is frankly materialistic. It is fortunate that there are many psycho-analysts who practise the Freudian technique without importing into it the virus of materialism.

The most important part of the work of Freud in the domain of *pure* psychology relates to the theory of complex formation in general, which has been elaborated by him. We shall give an account of this in the next chapter, not for the purpose of criticizing it, but in order to use it as the basis of our discussion of the materialistic complex. The principles and incidents of complex formation as enunciated by Freud furnish a satisfactory foundation for the elucidation of the materialistic complex by which Freud himself is affected. He has himself furnished the weapon which destroys the validity of the considerations which he puts forward in support of his materialistic philosophy. Such philosophy is worse than useless for therapeutic purposes. And it is difficult to see why he goes out of his way to preach materialism, except perhaps as a justification for the moral quicksands in which he finally leaves his patients to " find their own solutions ".

CHAPTER III

THE MATERIALISTIC COMPLEX

JUNG in his *Psychological Types*[1] distinguishes two essentially different types of mind—the introverted and the extraverted—differentiated by their attitude towards objective facts. The introvert's attitude to the object is an abstracting one—he endeavours to penetrate below the surface and seize upon the subjacent idea.

The extravert bases his decisions not upon subjective values but upon objective determinants. For his mentality there exists only the concrete and objective. His thinking is orientated by objective data transmitted through sense perceptions. Where subjective ideas come in they are such as have been acquired by tradition and by education. His moral point of view is conventional. In Jung's view thought is sterilised when thinking is mainly influenced by objective data, since it becomes " degraded into a mere appendage of objective facts, in which case it is no longer able to free itself from objective data for the purpose of establishing

[1] Translated by Dr. H. G. Baynes (Kegan Paul & Co.), pp. 412 *seq.*

an abstract idea". And Jung observes that "the materialistic mentality presents a magnificent example of this". In his view the materialist "conceives psychology as chemical changes taking place in the cell-ganglia, or as the extrusion and withdrawal of cell-processes or as an internal secretion," in fact, "reduces all mental phenomena to current physiological notions". Jung appears to regard Freud as belonging to the extraverted type and observes that "with Freud the basic formula is sexuality "—a position which Freud himself asserts.

Such in Jung's view is the type of mind which more readily lends itself to a materialistic bias, but the liability to the materialistic complex is by no means confined to this type. Let us consider the matter from the standpoint of complex formation in general.

The state of mind conditioned by a complex is one in which the person who is the subject of the complex has a prejudice more or less deeply rooted against the reception of any facts, opinions or beliefs which run counter to his "convictions". In more technical language a complex is a mental constellation fixed in the unconscious mind which opposes the reception of facts, opinions or beliefs which are in opposition to the complex. In its most legitimate form it is shown in that scientific scepticism

which holds at arm's length new facts and
theories which are in some way contrary to
previously accepted results, but keeping a final
judgment in suspense for the production of more
evidence. In its most acute phase the facts or
theories which run counter to the complex are
so disagreeable to the subject of the complex
that he absolutely rejects them, refuses to
examine the facts, readily accepts any evidence
or argument against them, however slight, but is
impervious to argument the other way, and, in
fact, has a mind completely closed even against
the mere consideration of the other side of the
case. Between these extremes are cases in
which the complex subsists more or less loosely
or acutely and in which there is more or less
possibility of the complex being broken down.
Familiar illustrations of political and sectarian
complexes will occur to the reader, where the
opinions of the subject on one side or the other
are rooted and inexpugnable.

It is in matters of opinion and belief, where
there are no crucial facts which can be taken
as settling the question that the effect of a
complex is most powerful. Its power is enhanced
by the fact that the complex is seated in the
unconscious mind and that its existence is
unknown to the subject. It rests upon feeling
and emotions, the intellect being rendered

subservient to and enlisted on the side of the emotion. It acts automatically in determining opinions without the knowledge of the subject, who is indeed powerless to determine his belief in opposition to the complex. Thus, suppose that a Protestant were asked to believe in transubstantiation in peril of the stake. Even under such a threat he would find it impossible to bring his mind to a genuine belief. His mental constellation would prevent it, however much he might desire it. History furnishes many such examples. Opinion and belief, in the absence of some compelling proof, are entirely determined by the complex, and in acute cases no proof would be compelling. Here then we are up against a phase of the human mind with which we have always to reckon. We have to guard against it in ourselves, we have to take it into account when considering the opinions of those who teach authoritatively, and it may be used as a friend or a foe in the education of children.

Freud and his pupils have thoroughly established the nature of complexes as above described and the principles on which complex formation depends.

It is curious that the principles of complex formation and the symptomatic results of a complex in stultifying and incapacitating

intellectual processes should emanate from Freud
and others who are themselves the subject of the
materialistic complex. They have been deduced
from the study of other complexes, but being of
general application they equally serve for the
elucidation of the materialistic complex. Undoubtedly those who formulated them little
suspected that they would be used to unravel
the materialistic complex by which they themselves were unknowingly affected. But for
this reason their enunciation is clear of any bias
for or against materialism.   A few citations from
the papers of Dr Ernest Jones[1], who is one of the
leading exponents of Freud in this country, will
indicate the general line on which they proceed.
He observes : " The large majority of conscious
mental processes in a normal person arise from
sources unsuspected by him " (p. 8).

" Although the importance of feeling in the
moulding of our judgments, beliefs and conduct
has for centuries been recognized by poets and
writers, academic psychology has usually allotted
to it a very subordinate position in relation to
what may be called the ' intellectual processes.'
Of late years, however, more and more recog-
nition has been given to the importance of
feeling ; until now one may fairly question
whether there exist any mental processes in

---

[1] *Papers on Psycho-Analysis*, Second Edition.

the formation and direction of which feeling does not play a part of the first rank . . .

" The causes of these mental processes are usually not only unsuspected by the individual concerned, but are repudiated and denied by him when the very existence of them is suggested. In other words, there exist elaborate psychological mechanisms the effect of which is to conceal from the individual certain feeling processes, which are often of the highest significance to the whole mind. The complexity and subtlety of these mechanisms vary with what may be called the extent of the necessity for concealment, so that the greater the resistance the individual shows to the acceptance of the given feeling the more elaborate is the mechanism whereby it is concealed from his consciousness."

One characteristic of concealment mechanisms in which the individual regards any enquiry into the source of the mental process as superfluous and explanation as non-existent, is " that the individual considers the given mental process to be self-explanatory and regards any further enquiry into its origin as being absurd, irrelevant, meaningless, unnecessary, and above all, fruitless. This, broadly speaking, is the mechanism that prevents the individual from becoming conscious of the source of the mental process " (p. 9).

" Summing up this class of mental processes, therefore, we may say that whenever an individual considers a given process as being too obvious to permit of an investigation into its origin, and shows resistance to such investigation, we are right in suspecting that the actual origin is concealed from him—almost certainly on account of its unacceptable associations. Reflection shows that this criterion applies to an enormous number of our fixed beliefs—religious, ethical, poetical and hygienic —as well as to a great part of our daily conduct " (p. 12).

In the class of cases in which the individual proffers an explanation of the mental process, but a false one, it is observed that everyone feels " that as a rational creature he must be able to give a connected logical and continuous account of himself, his conduct and opinions, *and all his mental processes* are unconsciously manipulated and revised to that end." Applying this, for instance, to the case of different sects holding divergent ideas as to religious doctrines, " there are a number of arguments used by each sect to support its special view of religion, and as a rule these are as convincing to the members of the given sect as they are unconvincing to members of other sects."

" The same arguments that with one man

proved so efficacious may be repeated (to another) with the most persuasive eloquence and are rejected with scorn as being obviously fallacious."

"It will be an interesting question for the future to determine how many of our most firmly held opinions are similar examples of the blind acceptance of the suggestive influence of our environment fortified by the most elaborate evasions and rationalizations."

Later it will be seen that all these observations of Dr Ernest Jones apply with great force to the materialistic complex.

Still more important in producing unconscious mentation are the complexes which are produced by repression. Repression is the exclusion of a pain-producing mental process from consciousness.

"In daily life this mechanism is extraordinarily frequent and shows itself in many ways, the simplest of which is the disinclination for being reminded of disagreeable occurrences which we would rather forget. There are many motives for this disinclination, the painfulness of an external situation being the least important; *more* important are such mental attitudes as shame, disgust, horror and the possibility of various internal thoughts and wishes."

"The manifestation of abnormally repressed

C

mental processes is to be understood only by consideration of the action of *intrapsychical conflict*. . . . Conflict between two tendencies or wishes results in a blocking and dissociation of the mental process concerned " (p. 23).

" There exist in the mind certain inhibiting forces which tend to exclude from consciousness all mental processes the presence of which would evoke there, either directly or by association, a feeling of ' unpleasantness '."

The term " exclude " may cover " on the one hand the expulsion from consciousness of an ' unpleasant ' mental process, or on the other the tendency to prevent the return of this to consciousness on any subsequent occasion."

Freud uses the term " censorship " to " cover the sum total of the repressing forces."

The repressing forces " guard consciousness as far as possible from the pain of disagreeable affects."

They " strive to prevent the complexes from entering consciousness " (p. 113).

" The conception of repression, as developed by Freud, is a purely hedonic one, the function of repression being exclusively to avoid pain " (p. 118).

" Processes occur in the unconscious which present all the attributes of mental ones except that the subject is not aware of them " (p. 121).

" The unconscious processes are of such a kind
as to be incompatible with the conscious ones
of the given personality, and are therefore
prevented from entering consciousness by the
operation of certain actively inhibiting ' repres-
sive forces.' The incompatibility in question
is most often of a moral order, the word moral
being taken in its widest possible sense. The
processes concerned then conflict with the
moral, social, ethical, modest or æsthetic standards that obtain in the person's consciousness ;
their very existence would be intolerable to him,
and he automatically refuses to acknowledge
to himself their presence in his mind " (p. 123).

Freud has applied these principles to explain
lapses of memory. After referring to this Dr.
Ernest Jones continues : " Most important,
however, is the extension of these principles in
the sphere of human judgment, for it is probable
that repressed complexes play as prominent a
part in distortion here as they do in minor
matters of memory mentioned above. On a
large scale this is seen in two ways—in the
minimum of evidence often necessary to secure
the acceptance of an idea that is in harmony
with existing mental constellations, or to reject
one that is incompatible with these. In both
cases it is often the affective influences rather
than intellectual operations that decide the

question. The evidence is construed quite differently when viewed in the light of one affective constellation from the way it is when viewed in the light of another " (p. 98).

Let us now apply these general principles to the consideration of the genesis and effect of the materialistic complex. In this complex the constellation of ideas which are repressed as having painful or disagreeable associations may include the notions of

Moral law and moral responsibility
God as the source of moral law
A future life
Free will

and similar ideas which fall naturally into the same constellation. Even the possibility of telepathy falls into the complex in the cases of Freud and Dr. Ernest Jones, the latter of whom suggests that a belief in telepathy is a " derivative of the flatus complex."

Let us now consider the various ways in which such a complex may be set up. Probably it is most readily and powerfully set up in the type in which strong sexual impulses come into conflict with powerful moral inhibitions. Dr. Ernest Jones remarks :

" The unconscious is the part of the mind which stands nearest to the primary instincts.

The unconscious is in a state of moral conflict with the standards of consciousness, for none of the other primary instincts is subjected to anything like the intensity of repression that the sexual one invariably is " (p. 122).

Now in the theory and practice of psycho-analysis many of the neuroses which come under the notice of the physician are attributed to repression of the sexual instincts. But the cases in which the sexual instincts have full play and the moral standards are repressed rarely come under the observation of the psychoanalyst. The fact that the outcome of the conflict may be, *not the repression of the sexual instincts, but of the moral standards*, hardly seems to have occurred to Freud and his exponents. Such a repression does not give rise to the symptoms of a neurosis, but it does give rise to definite psychological symptoms which are clearly recognisable. They do not affect physical health, but they affect the intellect and the logical faculty wherever these are applied to subjects which involve the element of morals, and they profoundly affect character. What these symptoms are can be fully gathered from the preceding extracts from the papers of Dr. Ernest Jones.

Let us trace out the course of such a conflict

a little more in detail. Our typical subject has
the ideas of a moral standard and moral responsibility implanted in him—let us say by education.
There comes a time when he has the impulse
to gratify sexual desires in the teeth of moral
standards. The outcome of the conflict is the
triumph of sexual instincts, and there arises at
the same time the disagreeable idea of a breach
of moral law. With repetition the sexual
impulse grows more over-mastering and the idea
of moral responsiblity fades away. It is too
painful to be entertained, and in the final outcome of the conflict the painful idea of moral
responsibility becomes repressed into the unconscious and with it the associated ideas of a
Divine law or a Divine law-giver. The idea
that a man is the creature of impulses and is not
really a free agent is easily attached to the complex and the further idea that to enjoy life is
the main thing and that there is no evidence
of a future life easily follows. All the ideas
associated with the notion of moral responsibility
become painful and the result of a conflict which
is worked out in this way is that the materialistic
complex is set up in its strongest form.

There are other ways in which the complex is
established, and it should be observed that it
is not necessary for a person to become a
libertine in order to set up the complex. But

it is clear that sexual licence, to a degree much less than that required to shock society, may co-operate with other circumstances to establish or to strengthen the complex. Human nature is prone to find excuses for its excesses, and the excuse that, after all, there may be no harm done and no such thing as moral responsibility, is likely to co-operate with other circumstances.

The education of a youth in materialism is, of course, one way in which such a complex may be acquired, and a materialistic outlook which is educational would naturally be strengthened in the manner above described, though in this case the conflict would be less, the resulting repression less formidable, and the complex probably less acute.

In this connexion it is germane to take into account the working of an authority complex and an anti-authority complex. Both these may be acquired in conjunction with some kind of parental complex which has probably been set up in early youth. A stern parent may give rise to an anti-authority complex in which there is an antagonism against the authority of the parent, which may be transferred by substitution and directed against a Teacher or Society or Divine Authority so that the child may become an anarchist or an infidel or in some other way temperamentally at war with authority of some or any kind. On the other hand the child may have a strong fixation upon a parent giving rise to an authority complex so that the ideas of the parent, be they materialistic or spiritualistic or strongly tinged with any form of sectarian religion, may become part of the mental constellation of the child.

A not uncommon way in which a materialistic complex may be acquired through early teaching deserves mention. A child may be brought up in the faith that the Bible is literally inspired and may accept ·the belief that the story of the swallowing of Jonah by the whale or the destruction of the walls of Jericho by the method described, or the standing still of the sun and moon at the command of Joshua, are historical incidents. He may be impressed with the belief that to question such incidents or the accuracy of any part of the Scriptures would destroy the foundations of religion. When he is a little older and has come under the influence of Biblical criticism or has acquired the scientific spirit, he will find the two sets of ideas confronting one another and in conflict, with the result that his early beliefs are overthrown. He has been taught that the things he now rejects were *fundamental*, and the result may easily follow that he rejects the whole set of religious ideas and becomes a materialist. It requires a lot of clear thinking to be able to separate what is really fundamental in religion from its accretions. An education such as has been described will inhibit such clear thinking, and if, as will often be the case, a conflict between sexual impulses and morals has already taken place, the ideas of religion will be the more easily repressed.

With the strict followers of Freud, who accept the whole of his teaching without reservation or criticism, the materialistic complex has merged into a Freudian complex. A professional complex of this kind fortifies the subjects of it against the acceptance of evidence or argument which runs counter to the complex. For these Freud has the infallibility of a Pope. Anyone who criticizes Freud is treated by them as outside the pale, and if possible, he is actually excluded from the Society to which Freud's worshippers belong. The attitude taken up is : " This is contrary to Freud and therefore it must be wrong ". They would like to reserve the designation " psycho-analyst " for those who have the Freudian complex. Unfortunately this is not possible, for a purely descriptive word cannot be a good trade-mark, even for the person who brings it to birth. It would be a good thing if the word did connote those who adopt Freud's moral standpoint so that they might be distinguishable. But unfortunately the word psycho-analysis (*pace* the Freudians) is accepted by all but the Freudians as meaning a method of analysing or disclosing the content of the unconscious mind for therapeutic purposes, without any necessary connection with the moral standpoint of Freud. Nothing is more desirable than that those who stand at the strict Freudian standpoint should have a distinctive name, so that they might not be confused with those whose views are not permeated by the materialistic virus.

The evidence of a complex is to be found, to use the words of Dr Ernest Jones, "in the minimum of evidence often necessary to secure the acceptance of an idea that is in harmony with the existing mental constellations, or to reject one that is incompatible with these". It likewise appears clearly in the feebleness of the argument by which a position in harmony with the complex is accepted and the vigour with which the contrary is repelled. It is shown in the want of logic which is used in the defence of a matter involved in the complex or in the rejection of a counter proposition. Furthermore, invective of a strength proportionate to the weakness of the logic, is common. It is displayed in the readiness with which some trivial matter is permitted to counter-balance matters of much graver import and in the facility with which excuses are made, putting altogether aside matters which run counter to the complex. It is shown in jumping to conclusions on nebulous bases, and in positiveness of assertion where conjecture only is possible.

The more acute symptoms of a complex which are well described by Dr Ernest Jones in the passages quoted above are distinctly pathological, that is to say, they indicate an unbalanced or disordered intellect, which is incapable of functioning properly on any subject which touches the complex. It may be compared with a delusion of a " person of unsound mind " which extends to a definite subject whilst the patient is perfectly sane in all other matters. The experience of the writer as a magistrate in the administration of the lunacy acts has been clear. Unless you are forewarned of the patient's delusion you may often talk with him for an hour on all sorts of subjects without getting any indications of dementia. But if you casually introduce the subject of the delusion the patient gives himself away at once. In the experience of the writer there are scientists of the highest intellectual capacity and the most trustworthy judgment on purely scientific matters who re-act acutely on any topic which runs counter to the materialistic complex.

They assume a position of superiority and of pity for the ignorance of one who holds a contrary opinion. They decline to consider seriously any contrary facts or evidence. Their attitude on the subject is the same as that of a physicist who might be asked to consider some new mechanical project for the attainment of perpetual motion without the expenditure of energy. He would (rightly enough) put the matter aside as one which was unworthy of serious consideration. But he would do it with an incontrovertible weight of evidence at his back. Our materialistic patient has a similar reaction against the ideas of God or free-will or human survival, but without any scrap of evidence to support assertions which he will nevertheless make as positively as if the doctrine of the conservation of energy were in question. The study of the materialistic complex throws light on this attitude of mind.

We have quoted above the opinion of Dr. Ernest Jones that the conflict between sexual impulses and moral standards is of the most intense kind. It follows that when the result of this conflict is the repression of the moral standards, the resulting materialistic complex is exceedingly powerful. Its intensity is such that its results may well be equivalent to those of a compulsion neurosis. He is obsessed by what we may call "compulsion ideas", which involve a real derangement of the mind. In a sense all ideas which find their roots in a complex instead of in fact or logic may be called "compulsion ideas". They may happen to be right or wrong, but if they are the result, not of reason and evidence but of a complex, they are still compulsion ideas. If the ideas are indubitably right the support of a complex may be all the better. But until we reach the stage of actual delusions it is difficult to find any compulsion ideas so powerful as those which spring from the materialistic complex. You may have a Tory or a Radical complex, a Baptist or an Anabaptist complex, but we find by experience that such complexes are often broken down. But in the case of a materialistic complex generated by such a conflict as above described, it would be hard to find instances of its dispersion. Of course we do not know the personal history of our scientists, who are materialistic propagandists, and the complex has different origins in different cases. In a recent article on "Human Survival" (*Hibbert Journal*, April, 1924),. the writer analysed one case of the materialistic complex, where there were distinct signs of a dispersal of this complex. But such cases are rare and it remains as a fact of experience that the materialistic complex in its acute stages is inexpugnable. The compulsion ideas which it carries with it are not always the same, but the following are some of those which are common :

Compulsion Ideas

1. There is no such thing as moral responsibility.
2. There is no survival after death. The mind ceases to exist when the physical brain is destroyed.
3. Free will does not exist. Our thoughts and actions are controlled by strict determinism.
4. There is no God and no such thing as spirit except as a function of matter.
5. There are no means of cognition other than the physical senses. Telepathy is non-existent.

Such are some of the chief compulsion ideas of the materialistic complex, but they are found in various combinations. Thus many are obsessed by 1 and 2, some add No. 3, fewer still add No. 4, Freud and his strict followers have the whole five, though there are signs that No. 5 is disappearing from Freud's complex.[1]

We shall consider the evidences of the complex in some of Freud's writings.

[1] See *Dreams and Telepathy* by Sigm. Freud (*International Journal of Psycho-analysis*, iii., 283).

CHAPTER IV

FREE WILL AND DETERMINISM

THE effect of the materialistic Complex is well illustrated by the psychological camouflage which Freud brings to bear on the subject of free-will in his *Psychopathology of Every-day Life*.[1] On the strength of certain matters occurring in every-day life in which he is able to show motivation from the unconscious mind when the will is inactive, he invites us to the generalization that *all* our thoughts and actions are the result of strict determinism and that our consciousness of free-will is an illusion. Here is a view which is so important and far reaching that one would have thought that a scientist would beware of cloaking a mere opinion under the guise of a proposition psychologically demonstrated. If Freud were able to convince the world that free-will is a mere illusion, that our choice of alternative actions was no real choice but the result of determinants which we could not control, the consequences would be incalculable. Yet he puts forward this proposition

[1] Translated by Dr. A. A. Brill (T. Fisher Unwin, Ltd.).

with a lack of evidence and of logic which only the materialistic complex can explain. Furthermore, Freud and his followers are not merely speculative philosophers. As psycho-analysts they deal with neurotic patients by revealing the complexes by which they are affected so as to give them a fresh start in life. What sort of a start can be founded on the underlying theory that a man cannot really help himself but is at the mercy of determinants over which he has no control ?

We must consider his " argument " a little more fully in order to appreciate its futility. This very futility—this acceptance of a logic which is clearly fallacious—is clear evidence of the complex. In this book, *The Psychopathology of Every-day Life*, Freud has shown how a number of actions in every-day life are regulated by determinants in the unconscious mind. For instance, he shows that the forgetting of a proper name (which we are apt to do from various causes) is often motivated by a repression caused by some unpleasant association which the remembrance of the name would bring to mind. He tells us he has analysed a large number of cases of forgetting, of which he gives in detail several, and finds that they usually lead to " intimate and painful things in the person analysed ". Referring to his own experiences he says (p. 38) : " When I analyse these cases of name forgetting occurring in myself, I find almost regularly that the name withheld shows some relation to a theme which concerns my own person and is apt to provoke in me strong and often painful emotions." And he gives a case in which he forgot a name which reminded him of a Vienna colleague, which touched his professional complex, and another in which he forgot the name of a station which reminded him of a sister and thus touched a " family complex ", of which he gives many illustrations. The " self reference " complex (personal, family or professional) he thinks is the most effective of the memory-disturbing complexes.

Blunders in speech, of which he gives various examples, are also shown to be motivated in the unconscious mind, and may often be traced to a half-repressed idea outside the intended context. So also as to mistakes in reading and writing, he holds that the same considerations apply and traces them to repressed elements of psychic life.

Referring to the forgetting of impressions and resolutions he says : " I shall report some striking examples of forgetting which for the most part I have observed in myself," and he concludes : " The forgetting in all cases is

D

proved to be founded on a motive of displeasure".
" Painful memories merge into motivated forgetting with special ease ".

With regard to " intentions ", the suggested
intention normally " slumbers in the person
concerned until the time for its execution
approaches. Then it awakes and excites the
action ". In cases in which the intention is not
carried out, Freud says : " I have found that
they could invariably be traced to some unknown
and unadmitted motives ", arising from some
antagonism in the unconscious. Many instances
are given, of which one must suffice. He
remarks : " In former years I observed that of
a great number of professional calls I only forgot
those that I was to make on patients whom I
treated gratis," which led him to make special
notes of calls. And he says : " I have invariably
found that intentions of some importance are
forgotten when obscure motives arise to disturb
them."

Freud explains on the same principle of
motivation from the unconscious various erroneously carried out actions (such as on arriving
at a friend's house pulling out one's own latch-
key instead of ringing the bell), or awkward
actions, apparently accidental but traceable to
an unconscious purpose in their execution. For
instance, Freud says : " Recently we passed

through a period in my house during which an unusual number of glass and china dishes were broken. I myself largely contributed to this damage. This little endemic was readily explained by the fact that it preceded the public betrothal of my eldest daughter. On such occasions it is customary to break some dishes and utter at the same time some felicitating expression ". And he gives many other cases of unintended actions motivated by unconscious intentions, such, for instance, as apparently accidental self-inflicted wounds which may really be the outcome of an unconscious intention to commit suicide.

Turning to the subject of " chance " actions which are executed idly and without any conscious intention, he finds that the determination of such action is really swayed by unconscious motives. Often the person is unaware of the chance action, such as playing with his watch-chain or jingling coins in his pocket which " regularly conceal sense and meaning to which other expression is denied ". The illustrations given are too long to quote, but they all involve the element of motivation from the unconscious.

Again, in the case of errors, Freud finds that they are determined by some repression or unconscious disturbing influence. Thus—to take

a short example : " A woman enquiring about a
mutual friend erroneously called her by her
maiden name. Her attention having been
directed to this error, she had to admit that
she disliked her friend's husband ". Freud also
gives illustrations of combined error and forgetting, also due to unconscious motivation.
Thus : " Jones left a letter for several days on
his desk, forgetting each time to post it. He
ultimately posted it, but it was returned to him
from the dead letter office because he forgot to
address it. After addressing and posting it a
second time it was again returned to him, this
time without a stamp. He was then forced to
recognise the unconscious opposition to the
sending of the letter ".

This is a short summary of the many illustrations given by Freud in the first 273 pages of his
book, which lead up to the final chapter
on " determinism — chance and superstitious
beliefs ". He gives further illustrations of
numbers and names apparently chosen by
chance, which, on analysis, proved to be motivated from the unconscious. And he concludes
generally that the common character of all such
faulty and chance actions as he has reviewed
" lies in the ability to refer the phenomena to
unwelcome repressed psychic material, which,
though pushed away from consciousness, is

nevertheless not robbed of all capacity to express itself ".

Such then are the materials upon which Freud bases the view that our lives are governed by strict determinism and that free will is non-existent. " Many persons ", says he, " argue against the assumption of an absolute psychic determinism by referring to an intense feeling of conviction that there is a free will ". But in his view this feeling is a delusion aud our " weighty and important decisions " are really due to " psychic compulsion ". But the deduction of his conclusions shows clear signs of the materialistic complex. For a careful review of all the many cases of faulty and chance actions (as Dr. Paul Bousfield was the first to note) shows that *in all cases the actions are determined without any active interference of the will. In every case the will is non-existent or is caught napping, and the act is determined by the content of the unconscious mind while the will slumbers.* Now to argue from cases *in which the will does not intervene,* that there is no such thing as free will, reveals a gap in logic which is one of the characteristics of the complex. For these cases only show that *in the absence of an effort of the will* determinism has free play.

The area in which determinism operates when the will is dormant is much more extended than that illustrated by chance and faulty actions. Nine-tenths of our lives are governed by determinism from the unconscious. All the habits of action and thought which we painfully acquire and which become rooted in the unconscious form determinants which are the background of every well-ordered life. We learn with effort to walk, to talk, to write. We acquire habits of thought, of self-control and of concentration. And this substratum of deterministic or automatic thought and action relieves us from conscious effort of will in most of the actions of daily life.   Here is a far wider ground of determinism than is illustrated by the narrow field of chance and faulty actions.

But it is obvious that this extended area of determinism, in which the will does not come into play, furnishes no argument against the operativeness of the will when it is used. All this useful determinism sets us free to grapple with things in which the will does come into play.   The fact that nine-tenths of our lives is automatically determined from the unconscious without voluntary effort cannot be used to show that in the remaining tenth of life the will is inoperative, except to a mind governed by the materialistic complex.   This materialistic complex, rooted in the unconscious, does indeed, in accordance with Freud's principles, lead to and is responsible for the opinion that there is no such thing as free-will. In accordance with the principles of complex motivation, the evidence of the nine-tenths is readily accepted as evidence for the remaining one-tenth, and the evidence of our own consciousness in favour of free-will is readily rejected. It should be carefully borne in mind that Freud's view as to the will is merely a pious (or impious) opinion which, as such, is necessarily motivated from the unconscious, which does undoubtedly determine mere opinions; that the feebleness of his logic is the clearest indication of a complex, and that in conjunction with similar opinions (to which we shall refer later) as to God and a future life, this complex may clearly be diagnosed as the materialistic complex. And the fact remains that psychology gives no real support to the view that the notion of free-will is illusory, whilst the experience of life is strong evidence to the contrary. The whole of this book is an elaborate camouflage so far as free-will is concerned, obscuring the subject by a mass of illustrations in none of which is there any effort of will.

CHAPTER V

TOTEM AND TABOO

IN his *Totem and Taboo* (Routledge) Professor Freud has investigated very minutely the elementary social and religious ideas of various primitive races all over the world. They display a striking similarity. Their essentials are akin among all the tribes and in all the countries to which he refers—Australia, New Hebrides, New Caledonia, New Britain, New Mecklenburgh, Fiji, Sumatra, The Barongas, Wakamba, Banks Island, Solomon Islands, Zulus, Basogus, Samojades in Siberia, Todus in S. India, Mongolians of Tartary, Tuaregs of the Sahara, Aino of Japan, Akamba and Nandi in Central Africa, Tinguanes in the Philippines, Nikobari Islands, Madagascar and Borneo. Freud tells us that "we can recognize in savage life a well-preserved stage of our own development" (p. 1). He has examined the psychology of primitive races by comparison "with the psychology of the neurotic as it has become known to us through psycho-analysis", and he finds the explanation of all "superstitions" in the compulsion ideas and hallucinations of neurotics.

48

In his *Psycho-pathology of Every-day Life,*
published five years previously, he had already
formulated an analogy between paranoiacs and
primitive man and said : " We venture to
explain in this way the myths of paradise, and
the fall of man, of God, of good and evil, of
immortality and the like . . . The gap between
the paranoiac's displacement and that of super-
stition is narrower than appears at first sight ".
Totem and Taboo must be regarded as a further
attempt to support this position and we find in
it also those logical gaps and that facile
acceptance or rejection of evidence which
characterizes the materialistic complex.

This wide area of primitive experiences does
no doubt furnish a legitimate field for generalization. There are certain incidents of taboo which
are found to be almost universal and upon which
Freud comments. It appears that among the
most primitive savages there were inherent in
the human race the ideas of
    1. Unseen beings such as we call spirits.
    2. A spirit in man which survives death.
    3. Elementary moral duties.
    4. Unseen powers whose anger was to be
       feared and whose protection might be
       afforded.

These notions were, of course, quite elementary
—perhaps as elementary as would have been

primeval man's notions of the multiplication
table. For instance, the ideas of demons or gods
or spirits are often indistinguishable, but the idea
of unseen powers is quite clear. The idea that
man has a spirit which survives is also plain.
The notions of morality which consist chiefly of
prohibitions against incest and against killing
are also quite definite. Elementary as they are,
to the savage mind these ideas represented
realities in the dim light of which they lived their
lives. In a gradually more evolved shape they
have represented realities for the greater part
of mankind ever since. It is upon those who
say that they always were delusions and therefore in their more developed form still are
delusions, that the burden of proof or of argument lies.

One would have thought that the existence of
these universal ideas in primitive times was
evidence to show that they corresponded to
psychic facts and that they were originally
implanted in the human mind as germinal ideas
capable of evolving with the physical and psychical evolution of man. But the weight of this
evidence is not even considered by Freud,
although the facts from which it is derived are
clearly recognized, as the following quotations
from *Totem and Taboo* will show.

Among all the numerous races whose customs

have been considered, " No race has yet been found without conceptions of spirits " (p. 152).

Taking the aborigines of Australia as the most backward and wretched of all the many tribes considered by him he remarks : " We surely would not expect that these poor naked cannibals should be moral in their sex life according to our ideas, or that they should have imposed a high degree of restriction upon sexual impulses. And yet we learn that they have considered it their duty to exercise the most searching care and the most painful rigour in guarding against incestuous sexual relations " (p. 2).

" It seems that the commandment, ' Thou shalt not slay ', which could not be violated without punishment, existed also among these savages, long before any legislation was received from the hands of a god " (p. 65).

Savages " do not conceal the fact that they fear the presence and the return of the spirit of a dead person " (p. 98).

" To primitive man the continuation of life— immortality—would be self-evident " (p. 127).

" The totem is regarded as the tribal ancestor of the clan, as well as its tutelary spirit and protector " (p. 3).

" Almost everywhere the totem prevails there also exists the law that the members of the same

totem are not allowed to enter into sexual
relations with each other ; that is that they
cannot marry each other. This represents the
exogamy which is associated with the totem "
(p. 6).

" Everybody descended from the same totem
is consanguineous, that is, of one family, and
in this family the most distant grades of relationship are recognized as an absolute obstacle to
sexual union " (p. 9).

" In Australia the regular penalty for sexual
intercourse with a person of a forbidden clan is
death " (p. 7).

The real sources of taboo " begin where the
most primitive and at the same time the most
enduring human impulses have their origin,
namely, in the fear of the effect of dæmonic
powers ".

The above quotations justify the statement
that after an exhaustive examination of savage
psychology as shown in all parts of the world, we
are entitled to draw from his findings the conclusion that elementary ideas of

         spirits
         survival
         morality
         and unseen powers

are present everywhere. We may further say
that the low development (for the most part)

of these ideas corresponds to the low mental and cranial organization of primitive man.

Now the origin of these ideas is unknown. Freud tells us :

" The totem exogamy makes the impression of a sacred statute, which sprang into existence no one knows how " (p. 14).

" The taboo prohibitions lack all justification and are of unknown origin " (p. 31).

" Both this word (taboo) and the system corresponding to it express a fragment of psychic life which is really not comprehensible to us " (p. 37).

" We do not know the origin of incest dread and do not even know how to guess at it " (p. 207).

It is clear, therefore, that theories as to the origin of these ideas are purely speculative. How they were generated or implanted in the primitive mind we do not know. Were they delusions comparable to those of neurotics according to Freud's theory ? Or were they implanted in the primitive mind by the same agency which is behind the physical evolution of man ? On the hypothesis that there is a supreme power in the Universe, according to whose plan evolution proceeds, it would follow that these elementary ideas were implanted in the race and have evolved *pari passu* with the physical and psychical advancement of the race. Furthermore, delusions concern themselves with objects and ideas familiar to the normal mind. The drunkard may see snakes, but snakes are real objects. His delusion does not invent snakes, it only imagines them where they are not. It is inconceivable how the savage mentality could have invented the idea of spirits— unseen intangible beings with mental attributes and powers. The theories of animism, according to which the forces of nature were supposed to be animated by unseen powers, do not really touch the difficulty. For the conception of an unseen and intangible power is a transcendental idea. Like begets like in the realm of ideas. You can feel the force of the wind and see its activities in a hurricane, but to attribute this to some spiritual power the idea of a Spirit must be there first. So remote is the idea of a spirit from anything in the realm of matter that it is difficult to see how it could arise spontaneously, even in connection with a hurricane. The idea of breath, wind, πνεῦμα, when once we have conceived of spirit, furnishes an easy analogy, but if primitive man had no idea of spirits, breath would be to him breath and wind, wind and nothing more.

Although the elementary ideas of spirits, survival, morality and unseen powers are admitted to be implanted in the primitive races of mankind, we shall not attempt to lay too much stress upon them. All that we postulate is that these primitive ideas *prima facie* correspond to realities and therefore the burden of proof that they are mere delusions rests upon those who put forward this view. Let us consider how Freud attempts to discharge this burden.

He tells us that the psycho-analyst " needs but a moment's reflection to realize that these phenomena are by no means foreign to him. He knows people who have individually created such taboo prohibitions for themselves. . . . If he were not accustomed to call these individuals ' compulsion neurotics ', he would find the, term ' taboo disease ' quite appropriate for their malady ". And the next sentence indicates the compulsion idea which is born of the materialistic complex. The psycho-analyst " *cannot resist* applying what he has learnt there to explain corresponding manifestations in folk psychology" (p. 44).

But the analytical mind of Professor Freud does furnish some resistance against the idea that the mentality of the neurotic is really comparable with the mentality of the primitive savage, although the resistance is not sufficient to overcome the influence of the complex. He

says : " There is one warning which we shall
have to give in making this attempt. The
similarity between taboo and compulsion disease
may be purely superficial. . . . We shall bear
this warning in mind, without, however, giving
up our intended comparison on account of the
possibility of such confusions ".

Let us take the first of his comparisons. He
has already told us that the taboo prohibitions
are of unknown origin and express a fragment
of psychic life which really is not comprehensible.

Now he says : " The first and most striking
correspondence between the compulsion prohibitions of neurotics and taboo lies in the fact
that the origin of these prohibitions is just as
unmotivated and enigmatic " (p. 45). There
are two gaps in this argument, even if the
analogy were admissible. First with compulsion
neurotics the origin of the compulsion idea is
often clearly discoverable by analysis. Secondly
he tells us that the origin of taboo prohibitions
is unknown, and he founds his " most striking
correspondence " on a double ignorance—ignorance of the motivation of compulsion neurosis,
and ignorance of the origin of taboo. How
these two unknowns can be elevated into a " most
striking correspondence " can only be explained
by the materialistic complex. You might as
well argue mathematically that if x and y are

both unknown quantities, therefore x = y.
We have not space to go through the less striking
correspondences, but the analogies will be found
to be equally superficial. Moreover, it is clear
that the main ideas of taboo do not lend themselves to the notion that they were generated by
something analogous to the origins of a compulsion neurosis. The ideas of spirits, survival,
sexual restriction and unseen powers, universal
as Freud finds them to be, and scattered all over
the world, point to a common origin. It would
be a marvel if the sporadic generation of chance
delusions independently in places as far apart
as the poles, should have resulted in this uni-
formity of primitive belief and morality. These
common psychic features of widely-scattered
races are just as much fundamental features as
the common cranial and physiological features
of the widely-scattered human family. It is
far more rational to suppose that these common
ideas express universal realities in a crude form
suitable to the stage of evolution to which they
belong, than that they are mere sporadic
delusions. And the real truth is that scientific
psychology has nothing to say to the contrary.

We do not propose to follow all the conclusions
which Freud derives from his comparison with
compulsion neurotics. Conscience, says Freud,
" is the inner perception of objections to definite

E

wish impulses ", but says he : " one may
venture the assertion that if the origin of guilty
conscience could not be discovered through
compulsion neurotic patients, there would be no
prospect of ever discovering it " (p. 116). None,
indeed, for the materialist ! " Spirits and
demons were nothing but the projection of
primitive man's emotional impulses " (p. 153).
" Psycho-analytic investigation of the individual
teaches with especial emphasis that God is in
every case modelled after the father—and that
God at bottom is nothing but an exalted father "
(p. 244). Perhaps there is a vestige of truth in
this idea of the disordered mind of the neurotic ! !
And he finally observes (p. 260) : " I want to
state the conclusion that the beginnings of
religion, ethics, society and art meet in the
Œdipus complex. This is in entire accord with
the findings of psycho-analysis, namely that the
nucleus of all neuroses as far as our present
knowledge of them goes is the Œdipus complex ".
Alas for religion and ethics ! Alas for society
and art ! " A process like the removal of the
primal father by the band of brothers must have
left ineradicable traces in the history of mankind " (p. 25). And so this parricidal impulse,
this " guilty deed of primordial times ", " this
great event of man's primal history ", is the real
source of religion, ethics, society and art ! !

And after all, the notion that primeval races were generally accustomed to kill off the father, is a pure speculation, with only the most trifling evidence to support it. Furthermore, the evidence that *normal* people in general are affected by the Œdipus complex is scanty, and the conclusion that " religion, ethics, society, and art " sprang from the mentality of neurotics is not likely to be accepted by normal people.

We must always bear in mind that the generalizations of psycho-analysis are founded on the study of abnormal minds. It is clear from the perusal of Freud's writings that his mentality is abnormal. Much of his psychology is drawn as one would expect from the study of his own mind, but most of it from the analysis of his patients. For instance, the Œdipus complex is one very frequently found—so much so that Freud suggests that it is " the nucleus of all neuroses ! " In his *Psycho-pathology of Every-day Life* Freud was dealing chiefly with the mentality of normal people from which it was legitimate to generalize. But there is no justification for extrapolating from the mentality of neurotic patients to that of normal people and even less for carrying the extrapolation on to the primitive minds of primeval savages. The way in which this analogy is used by Freud throughout *Totem and Taboo* must be taken as an illus-

tration of the facility with which weak evidence
and feeble argument are marshalled in favour of
materialism by a person who is the subject of the
complex. The burden of proof that these
primary ideas—spirits, survival, morality and
unseen powers—were delusions, is upon the
materialist, and it is clear upon a perusal of
Totem and Taboo that this burden has not been
discharged, and that the assertion that psychology proves these ideas to be myths is unfounded.

Little harm is done so long as it is recognized
that these theories which the subject of the
materialistic complex so lightly adopts are but
personal opinions born of the complex and have
no foundation in psychological facts. But no
normal man, without the complex, can regard
them as leading to the conclusion that ideas of
spirits, survival, morality and unseen powers are
mere "superstitions". Psychology does not
furnish any data upon which such conclusions
can be logically based.

CHAPTER VI

LOVE—'Αγάπη—AMOR

To get a clear insight into typical differences it is often useful to look at the two extremes. On the one hand we find the entirely selfish and sensual type, in all respects self-seeking—its own pleasure, or profit—quite regardless of the feelings of others. It even sinks below the brute type—as for instance in the case of the man who combines cruelty with selfishness and beats and starves his own wife and children. On the other hand we have the type described by St Paul, whose characteristic is 'Αγάπη (charity, as it is translated)—a love for others which is regardless of self. The typical example of this type is Christ. Between these extremes and generally far from either is to be found the majority of the human race.

A materialistic psychology is inclined to look upon the Christ type as neurotic. As to this attitude Jung remarks : " The views advanced from time to time from the psychiatric side concerning the morbidity of Christ's psychology are nothing but ludicrous rationalistic twaddle, altogether remote from any sort of comprehension of the meaning of such processes in the history of man ".[1]

Whence comes the tendency to regard the Christ type as neurotic ? Simply because it will not fit into Freud's sex formula. It can only be brought into the range of sex phenomena by regarding it as pathological. Newton's corpuscular theory of light held the field until one phenomenon was discovered with which it was inconsistent. Then the undulatory theory of light and the luminiferous ether came to birth and displaced the corpuscular theory. The existence of the Christ type is the fact which will not fit into Freud's theory. Hence the theory of a psychology wholly based on sex corpuscles must give way to a psychology which recognises the more ethereal psyche as one of the two components of human nature. If the psyche were but a function of the soma the sex formula would be right. But the dual view of human nature opens up a very different prospect. As soon as we regard the psyche and the soma as differing in kind—the soma as the mere temporary vehicle of the psyche—we can differentiate at once between those characteristics which belong essentially to the psyche, those more transitory characteristics which mark the con-

[1] *Psychological Types*, p. 71.

nection of psyche and soma, and those further characteristics which are essentially somatic. We shall then no longer degrade the attribute of love, which is essentially of the psyche to the level of the sexual impulses which are an attribute of the soma.

A sound psychology must inevitably take into account those highest manifestations of love which experience tells us are independent of somatic or erotic impulses. The experience of mankind as recorded in history is not to be dismissed by neurotic analogies. Unfortunately we have no completely distinctive word for this emotion. The word love has so many somatic connotations that it has ceased to be distinctive. We shall therefore make an artificial use of the word *amor* to distinguish this altruistic emotion just as Freud has used the word *libido* in an artificial way. Unfortunately the word " charity ", which is used in St Paul's sublime description of this emotion, has also other connotations. But St Paul's description of 'Ἀγάπη which is translated " charity ", will serve as our definition of amor, which we will use for the purposes of this chapter.

" Though I bestow all my goods to feed the poor and though I give my body to be burned and have not *amor*, it profiteth me nothing."

" *Amor* suffereth long and is kind, *amor*

envieth not, *amor* vaunteth not itself, is not
puffed up—seeketh not her own, is not easily
provoked, thinketh no evil—beareth all things
—endureth all things, *Amor* never faileth."
Here is a description of an emotion, which,
though in its highest manifestations it is rare,
yet must be taken account of by psychology.
The existence of the emotion which we call *amor*
in some of the best and noblest of the human
race is a psychic fact.   In its highest form it
was exemplified in the life of Christ.   It is still
exemplified in rare members of the human race.
It is a psychic quality which has to be reckoned
with.   Now Freud reduces this to the level of a
somatic quality.   Nor does he even regard it
merely as an extension of sexual impulses, but
bases it on their perversion.   " The beginnings
of religion, ethics, society and art meet in the
Œdipus Complex.   This is in entire accord with
the findings of psycho-analysis, namely that the
nucleus of all neuroses as far as our present
knowledge of them goes is the Œdipus Complex."[1]   Such are the conclusions to which we
are led by regarding the psyche as a mere
function of the soma.

Unless we regard *amor* as a distinctly psychic
characteristic we fail to give a coherent account
of the whole of human nature.   It is true that

[1] *Totem and Taboo*, p. 260.

amor—the love that seeketh not its own, that loves humanity as itself—is only exemplified in comparatively few members of the race. But that is no reason why psychology should ignore it or classify it as a sexual emanation. Those in whom it exists are the salt of the earth. They are in the forefront of psychic evolution. Like the few outstanding musicians, poets and painters they stand out from the crowd. The fact that *amor* is the characteristic of a few does not detract from, but enhances, the importance of recognizing its psychic as distinct from its somatic quality. It represents the highwatermark of the advancing tide of civilization. It has given birth to the ideals of social service which are springing up. It is on these ideals. and their expansion that we have to rely to hold in check and overcome the ideas of class warfare which threaten to overturn such civilization as we have reached.

The notions of class warfare are the very antithesis of *amor*. They are the outcome of the primitive somatic instincts, whilst *amor* at its best is purely an outcome of our highest psychic instincts.

It might be suggested that altruism was much the same thing as amor. But this is not so. Altruism rather implies a philosophic or intellectual outlook, and lacks the emotional element which characterises *amor*. Amor involves a determinant which diverts psychic energy towards the attainment of its selfless objects. Of course both altruism and amor are the exact opposites of selfishness, but amor is a constantly active opponent. Selfishness is a somatic instinct, the primitive form of which was the seizing and appropriating of food. In Amor, which seeks to give and not to take, we find nothing of the primitive somatic instinct. The instincts of maternity seem akin to amor, but they have a limited field of exercise, whilst of *amor* it may be said, *nihil humani me alienum puto*, and even this is too narrow, for the ambit of amor extends beyond the human race.

Psychologists necessarily draw much of their psychology from introspection and the examination and analysis of their own experiences and mentality. If you were to ask some psychologists for some information as to the incidents of telepathy they would deny its existence or reply in the language of one of Freud's followers that " a belief in telepathy is a psychological development of the *flatus complex* ". So the emotion amor does not fall within the range of common experience, and if you were to ask some psychologists as to this emotion—a love that seeks to benefit others and is regardless of self—they might reply that they had no experience of such an emotion, that they had never come across it, or that it was a psychological derivative of the Œdipus complex. But there is too much evidence for telepathy to allow it to be disposed of so easily. And there is too much historical evidence of the psychic reality of the emotion which we have called *amor* from the days of Christ and St. Paul down to the present time to allow a normal person, unaffected by the materialistic complex, to doubt its existence. There are living examples of those who have given their lives to the service of humanity, and it is too much to ask us to believe that the love of mankind which activates them is the sublimated dregs of an abnormal sexuality. Their love and their energy cannot be held to spring from somatic roots but belong to the psychic plane. We have enlarged upon *amor* partly as an example of those psychic attributes which are clearly non-somatic, and partly because Freud, with the primary somatic instincts ever before him in his constant contact with neurotics whose maladies he traces to sexual origin, has dragged amor down from a psychic to a somatic level. There are other human attributes, such as the musical faculty which belong to the psychic and not to the somatic plane, but we must be content with the endeavour to place amor and energy on the higher level. To the consideration of energy we next proceed.

CHAPTER VII

ENERGY

A DEFECT of Freud's psychology which involves serious consequences is the confusion of sexual energy with psychic energy, and the attribution to sexual forces of that which belongs to man's higher nature. It may be true, as Freud says[1] that " sexual impulses have contributed invaluably to the highest cultural, artistic and social achievements of the human mind ". But unless in conjunction with the diviner impulses of the human mind the sexual impulses would have left us wallowing. The energy displayed as the outcome of amor, philanthropic Love, or unselfishness is, according to Freud, a transmuted form of sexual energy. The sexual forces, he says, are " sublimated, that is to say, their energy is turned aside from its sexual goal and diverted towards other ends, no longer sexual and socially more valuable ".[2] But, says he : " there is a danger that a rebellion of the sexual impulses may occur against this *diversion of*

[1] *Lectures*, p. 17.   [2] *Loc. cit.*, p. 17.

their energy ". From these and other passages it is clear that Freud regards sexual energy as the source of the energies of man's higher nature. Sexual energy is to be sublimated—diverted from its natural channel—to form an energy fund for other ends " socially more valuable ". But there have been noble characters whose unselfish love and efforts for humanity refuse to be classified as the result of a mere diversion of sexual energy. For all we know such people may have expended their sexual energy in a normal way. Are we to conclude that the " sublimation " of the remainder of their sexual energy accounted for the fund of philanthropic energy which they displayed ? The fact is that Freud's theory fails to account for such people, who must draw their psychic energy from a higher source than the dregs of sexual energy.

From the energy point of view we can easily recognize two distinct and extreme types. On the one hand we have men who have an excess of physical energy which is expended in physical activity, but who are intellectually inert. At the other extreme we have men who are intellectually full of energy and activity but whose physical energy is at a very low ebb. No doubt the highest type is both physically and psychically active, and the proper direction of physical energy often absorbs a large amount of psychic energy, but the extremes help us to see that the two kinds of energy are distinct, and the intermediate cases suggest that the relative amounts are often very different.

Psychic energy we should characterize as the mental energy which accompanies thought. Some thoughts are merely idle. They flit across the field of consciousness without any energy component. They are not purposive. They do not tend to lead to action. They may be reminiscent, they may be telepathic, but they are only transient. We are not conscious of their origin and they take their departure unheeded. On the other hand some thoughts are inspiring. They may come from the unseen, they may be telepathic, or derived from books lectures, conversation or otherwise. They bring an access of psychic energy and we do well to entertain them, to consolidate them as it were, to elaborate their outlines, to exploit them for all they are worth and to let the imagination play upon them until their fruitful ideas sink into the unconscious—charged with psychic energy and ready to become the springs of action. It is not easy to say how psychic energy is absorbed, but experience tells us that there are some thoughts so charged with beneficent energy that we feel as if a new impetus had been given to us together with a fund of energy available in a given direction. When Newton saw the apple fall from the tree (if the story be true, which matters not for the purpose of illustration) the idea suggested bore fruit in the theory of universal gravitation and unravelled the mechanics of the solar system. Whether the idea jumps into the mind charged with energy from without, or whether the play of the imagination on the idea diverts psychic energy upon it, it is clear that such an idea sinks into the mind with a charge of energy. Freud speaks of the " libido " repressed into the unconscious as " a force at work in the mind ". We are equally entitled to speak of a potent idea which sinks into the mind as " a force at work in the mind ". But the " force " or the energy with which it works is not somatic but psychic.

On the other hand some thoughts are mischievous. We may not be able to prevent their ingress, but if we entertain them and let the imagination play upon them they involve a mischievous diversion of psychic energy. We cannot control their ingress but we can ensure their rapid expulsion and so prevent the mischievous diversion of psychic energy which their entertainment involves. To let the imagination play upon them, to consolidate the ideas which they carry, is to ensure that these mischievous ideas will sink into the unconscious, charged

with a psychic energy which will inevitably tend
to their exploitation.

According to the materialistic hypothesis,
psychic energy is indistinguishable from somatic
energy. It holds that thought is a kind of
secretion of the brain, due, it is supposed, to the
metabolism of the grey matter, and therefore
in the ultimate a product of the food which we
eat. Hence it is not surprising that no distinction is drawn between somatic and psychic
energy. But whatever our conception of psychic
energy may be there can be no doubt about what
we mean by somatic or physical energy. The
doctrine of the conservation of physical energy
is clear. We cannot create such energy, we can
only use it. Its source can be traced to the sun,
and all the food we eat and the coal we burn in
our steam boilers import so much physical energy
derived from the sun. But neither physiologists
nor psychologists have been able to show that
physical energy can be turned into psychic
energy and that the doctrine of the conservation
of energy can be made to include both. In fact,
careful calorimetric experiments have shown
that the psychic energy employed (say) in
solving a mathematical problem does not involve
any consumption of physical energy.

The notion that ideas charged with energy
can be included in the doctrine of the conser-

vation of energy has no experimental foundation. It is therefore rational to draw as shapr a distinction between somatic energy and psychic energy as we draw between matter and ideas. What may be the source of psychic energy or the psychic mechanism by which it is absorbed and utilized is a matter of speculation. We are not sufficiently behind the scene to envisage it. But as a mere speculation we may surmise that the food of the mind consists largely of ideas which carry an energy charge. Some of these ideas may come to us telepathically, some from books, lectures or our environment in general. Whether such a speculation be right or wrong does not affect the distinction which we seek to draw between physical and psychic energy. To absorb the full energy which ideas charged with energy can impart, the mind must dwell upon them and assimilate them.

Now according to Freud the energy behind the sex instincts is about the only kind of energy at man's disposal. Man for him is an animal with a more highly developed cerebral and nervous organization. The notion that man differs from lower animals in the possession of a psyche which will persist, which is not a function of the brain, and of which the brain is merely an instrument, and that this psyche has psychic instincts and psychic energy which differentiate

F

man from the mere animal with its physical instincts and energy is not dreamt of in his philosophy. (For after all it is philosophy, and psychology can teach us nothing to the contrary in this matter, though Freud covers his philosophy with a psychological camouflage). According to Freud the sexual instincts with their " libido " are not only the nucleus of all neuroses but of man's higher nature.

We have seen that he says : " The beginnings of religion, ethics, society and art all meet in the Œdipus complex ", as a generalization from the mentality of the neurotics whom he has found afflicted with this complex. In his view the energy which springs from the sexual instincts is psychic energy and it is the sublimation or diversion of sexual energy which is the aim. According to the present view the desideratum is *to prevent the flow of psychic energy into erotic channels*. To make the matter clearer let us define the terms we use. Let us call the energy of the physical impulses of the sexual instincts by the name of sexual energy. When the imagination has been brought into play so as to divert psychic energy into sexual channels, we may call this reinforced sexual energy by the name of erotic energy. Let us call the energy of thought and imagination which is employed in channels which have no sexual components psychic energy pure and simple. We may illustrate the three kinds of energy.

1. Sexual energy as we see it exemplified in animal life is called forth by physical stimuli of smell, sight and other sensory factors. We do not credit a dog, or at all events a worm, with thinking erotically, but the occasion of the physical stimuli is sufficient to call the latent sexual energy into full activity. Without this physical stimulus the sexual energy is dormant.

2. Erotic energy is the outcome of thought and imagination. When the imagination is allowed to play on sexual matters, the sexual energy is reinforced by a diversion of psychic energy into physical channels, and the sexual energy so re-inforced takes on the form which we call erotic energy.

3. As an example of pure psychic energy we may take the case of Eliezer ben Yehudah, which is fully described in Chapter VIII.

Every normal person is conscious of a certain amount of psychic energy, just as he is conscious of a certain amount of physical energy. The source of the latter can be traced to the sun. It may either be used or misused. So psychic energy must come from a source outside, and this energy also may be either used or misused. Day by day we require to appropriate a ration of psychic energy if we wish to maintain a healthy psychic activity.

Different people absorb supplies of psychic energy in different ways. Probably the energy we absorb depends largely upon our outlook on life, upon the ideals which we cherish and upon the ideas which we absorb from our environment. Having then a store of both kinds of energy at our disposal, how is its utilization determined? The answer is that the will operates the sluice gates by which either form of energy can be turned into appropriate or inappropriate channels.

Psychic energy may be used to further non-sexual aims—all that constitutes the life of a man apart from the sexual, which latter should form a very small fraction of his existence. But if the imagination is allowed to play upon sexual matters this psychic energy will provide a fund of erotic energy which may be repressed in the conflict with moral standards with possible pathogenic results, or overflow the barrier of moral standards and become the nucleus of a materialistic complex.

According to Freud erotic conditions may result in " sexual toxins ". In his view certain pathological analogies " necessitate our regarding the neuroses as the effect of disturbances in the sexual metabolism, due either to more of these sexual toxins being produced than the person can dispose of, or else to internal and even mental conditions which interfere with the proper disposal of these substances."[1]

But analogy also suggests that the emotion accompanying the generation and accumulation of erotic energy is responsible for the secretion of these toxins, and that a normal man who did not allow his psychic energy to be diverted by the imagination into erotic channels would escape this sexual " intoxication ".

It seems clear that the way to avoid the generation of erotic energy and the secretion of " sexual toxins ", is to prevent the play of the imagination on erotic subjects. The man who looks at another eating a lemon will almost certainly experience an abnormal secretion of saliva. And the man who indulges in erotic imaginings will equally certainly experience an access of erotic energy. We are not here in the realm of hypothesis but of experience. If the imagination is allowed to run riot on sexual matters, it is a matter of experience that erotic energy is generated.

Thus it will be seen that Freud's notion of the sublimation of erotic energy entirely leaves out of account the fact that control of the imagination will prevent the generation of erotic energy.

[1] *Lectures*, p. 234.

Here then is the point at which the sluice-gate
must be shut against the diversion of psychic
energy if a healthy equilibrium is to be main-
tained. This does not involve repression.
Pathogenic repression comes in when erotic
energy has been stored up by a diversion of
psychic energy through an unbridled imagination
to such an extent that it would break bounds
if not repressed. For a normal man the prevention of this diversion of psychic energy is not
difficult. It should be fully utilized in non-
sexual channels. An objectless mind is an easy
prey to erotic imagination. But a steadfast
habitual barring of the door leading to lower
channels is necessary. Whenever erotic thoughts
emerge and the imagination begins to play upon
them, they must be sharply dismissed. To
secure this some formula should be decided on
which may be mentally repeated and which is of
such a nature as to give an entirely new turn to
thought. It must be of a forceful kind which
shall draw its own train of associations with it
and of a wholly different character. A pithy
motto or text or verse which shall have the power
of leading to a new and captivating or strenuous
chain of thought should be decided upon and
always used when the occasion arises, and so
prevent the diversion of psychic energy into the
erotic channel. One of the most baneful ways

of increasing erotic energy by pyschic diversion is the reading of novels which deal with sex problems. That the reader in imagination enters into the part of the hero (or villain) may be often perceived by the stimulation of physical phenomena. But whether this be so or no, such literature, unless it disgusts the reader, inevitab'y causes a diversion of psychic energy into sexual channels. The sex problem literature is certainly responsible for many of the actual sex problems of life. Any one who wishes his sexual life to be normal and easily controlled should avoid such literature like the plague. When plays or books pass beyond a certain point of indecency they are controlled by the censor or the courts. But if a censorship of books.which do not reach this point but are sexually mischievous, were in force, so that every book of this character were required to be printed with a black border on the title page or the cover, a warning would be given which would enable the reader who desired not to be burdened with an excess of sexually directed energy to avoid it. Licentious conversation and all other modes of setting the imagination at work in this direction should, of course, equally be avoided. The whole point is that the control of thought and imagination so that psychic energy may not be diverted into sexual channels will prevent an

excess of erotic energy which will be a burden
and require suppression or outlet.

How far these psychological facts can be
utilised in treatment where an actual neurosis
has been set up must be a matter for the psycho-
therapist in the individual case having regard to
the idiosyncrasies revealed by analysis or otherwise. But Freud's general dictum seems quite
inappropriate. By analysis he endeavours to
bring the repressions into consciousness so that
" the pathogenic conflict is exchanged for a
normal one which must be decided in one way
or another ". And at this stage " the analyst
refrains from playing the part of mentor. He
wants the patient to find his own solutions for
himself ". And the kind of solution which may
present itself may be gathered from his observation in the case of the woman brutally treated
by her husband who may develop a neurosis
" if she is too cowardly or too conventional to
console herself secretly with another man ".
Of course a materialist may regard freedom from
neurosis at the expense of character as being
worth while. But on our hypothesis, according
to which character survives, it is not worth
while.

One would have thought that instruction as
to the way in which, by giving reins to the
imagination, erotic energy may be increased to

such a point that either character or health will suffer, might be an important element in curative treatment in some cases. But the fact that control of the imagination may prevent the generation of erotic energy is not mentioned by Freud. The reason must be that, denying the dual constitution of man he regards all erotic energy as a primary product which has to be dealt with, whilst he fails to perceive that excess of erotic energy is a secondary product due to the work of the imagination in diverting psychic energy into physical channels. It appears to us that this is one of the major defects of the Freudian psychology which arises directly from a materialistic view of human nature. To regard the psychic energy of the mind as a sublimated form of " libido " or erotic energy is an error of the first magnitude.

CHAPTER VIII

WILL-POWER

OUR consciousness of a will free to select alternatives and to motivate the pursuit of a chosen path of conduct is a psychic fact. Unless this consciousness can be shown to be a delusion, which Freud has failed to do, we must accept the fact of free-will and act upon it. This is not to say that powerful determinants, chiefly motivated by the pleasure principle, may not act against the will and often overbear it. But in any such conflict we must recognize that the will is one of the determinants.

What is the will ? The answer cannot be put into the form of a definition. If one put the question : What is thought ? no definition would encompass the idea. Will and thought are elementary conceptions arising out of our own psychic experiences. When the Self is asserted in opposition to some resistance or inertia we are conscious that the will is acting. We are conscious of thinking. We are conscious of willing. Both ideas stand on the footing of an experience of consciousness.

We often speak of " will-power ", but it should be borne in mind that the will is probably a directing agency and not really a source of energy. We speak of the " horse-power " of an engine or a motor car, by which we mean merely that the engine is so organized that if energy be supplied from without (by coal or petrol) the engine can exert a given amount of power.

So when we speak of greater or less " will-power " we mean that the individual is so organized as to be able to utilize efficiently more or less psychic energy. The will-power of individuals varies enormously. But even where the will-power is very weak it is possible to supplement it greatly in the manner to be pointed out. Where the will-power is great and the supply of psychic energy is abundant, we have men of great achievements for good or ill. When we look at historical examples of great achievements carried through in the face of great obstacles our common sense (which we must not surrender at the bidding of psychologists) tells as that " the unconquerable will and courage never to submit or yield " is something that we must not look upon as a mere hallucination.

We have already pointed out that the source of psychic energy must be regarded as external to the individual. It seems as unscientific to regard the individual himself as a generator of psychic energy as it would be to regard him as a generator of physical energy. Somehow he absorbs psychic energy as he absorbs food, and some people have a vastly greater amount of psychic energy at their disposal than others. But the will may clearly be regarded as a directive agent for this energy. When we hold in our hands the nozzle of a hose pipe, through which a stream of water is flowing, the energy is in the water, the nozzle is an instrument for directing it. Or, to take another analogy, a ship is propelled through the water by the energy of the steam in the engines generated by the fuel under the boiler, but it is the rudder which directs the course of the ship against winds and currents and in the neighbourhood of shoals and rocks. So we may regard the will as one determinant of the channel through which energy flows or as the rudder by which the individual steers the human ship in the face of psychic shoals and rocks or in the teeth of winds and counter currents.

It is the national will which enables a nation to carry through a conflict in the face of discouragements and disasters to ultimate victory. This is but the integration of all the wills of individuals, even though this includes a minority of pacifists. It is the individual will which enables a man in the face of opposition and hope deferred to bring to fruition great ideas or to initiate and carry through great movements to a successful issue. In the face of scores of examples which might be given it seems idle to deny the efficacy of the will as the director of great enterprises requiring not merely an unfailing supply of psychic energy but a persistent direction of this energy towards the objective.

It will not be out of place to give an example of this will-power which overcomes all obstacles and breaks down all opposition, which will be more striking than any comment. For this purpose we reproduce from *The Times* of 1st January, 1924, an account of the life work of Eliezer ben Yehudah from the pen of its correspondent at Jerusalem.

"THE REVIVAL OF HEBREW.

" At the time of writing the whole of Palestine Jewry is marking the first anniversary of the death of Eliezer ben Yehudah, who died in December, 1922. The achievement and personality of this man are remarkable enough to deserve the attention of a far wider circle than just Palestine and the Jews.

" After the Babylonian Exile Hebrew all but died ; it was revived in Maccabean times to a certain extent, but after the Fall of Jerusalem

in A.D. 70 it ceased to be a spoken language ;
the linguistic powers of the Jews, notorious in
all ages, enabled them quickly to acquire the
language of their adopted place of exile and
Hebrew ceased to exist except as the literary
medium of a handful of scholars and as the
liturgical language of the Synagogue.

" It was at this stage that there came to the
Holy Land a young man, aged about 25, with no
means, no fame, no influential backing, and
not even a moderately healthy constitution.
He possessed but one thing—a will-power at
which one stands aghast. He chose to exert
this power in one direction : to revive the
Hebrew language, which had lain dead nearly
twenty centuries ; to equip it fully with all the
resources of an ordinary living speech, and to
habituate his fellow-Jews to the use of this
language in every department, public and
private, of their lives. And this purpose he
achieved to the fullest extent.

" With the accomplished fact before our eyes,
it is by no means easy to appreciate rightly all
the obstacles which have been overcome. A
few, however, we can realise. He had to cope
with a race which admittedly is the most
obstinate in creation. When Ben Yehudah
came to Palestine in 1881 the 50,000 Jews he
found here were all ' Orthodox ', leading their

lives strictly in accordance with the complicated religious code ; and to these Jews Hebrew was ' the Holy Language ', the language of Scripture and of Prayer. To use it for any other purpose was a blasphemous profanation. Ben Yehudah came, and, metaphorically, shaved his face, blacked his boots, and blew his nose in Hebrew, Ben Yehudah was, therefore, ostracized, anathematized, ' cut off from the congregation '. He must bury his own dead children as best he could ; his brother European Jews refused to touch his dead wife and take her to the Mount of Olives ; the religious leaders denounced him to the Turkish authorities on a trumped-up charge of preaching treason in a newspaper article, and Ben Yehudah spent some months in a foul Turkish gaol.

"Yet that astonishing will-power still stood firm. He refused to speak any language but Hebrew ; the Jews around him, entering Palestine in increasing numbers from all parts of the world, spoke almost every language under the sun except Hebrew (though Yiddish, a Jewish-German jargon, the language of Whitechapel, predominated), but his persistent combativeness in the end made others speak Hebrew, too. He edited newspapers, he organized societies, he taught in schools till he infected others with his own enthusiasm. He raised up children of his

own and made them talk Hebrew from the
cradle. His ideals spread gradually from family
to family, until, unit by unit, a generation arose
in Palestine which knew no language but
Hebrew.

" MODERN NEEDS.

" And so his life passed for 41 years in Jerusalem. He was untiring, spurring and goading
on the half-hearted, allowing them no rest,
volcanically eruptive under pressure of opposition, tireless in seeking out new openings,
adamant against allowing any concession, single-
minded with all the irresistibility of single-
mindedness, seeing only one object in life—that
his people should speak the language of their
forefathers in their ancient land.

" But there was another, in some respects
a more drab, side to the attainment of his ideal.
A language disused in current speech some 2,000
years needs more than enthusiasm to recreate it.
A language that could serve to express the ideas
and voice the needs of the last century B.C. was
helpless when confronted with the ideas and
needs of the 19th century A.D. Here again the
will of this remarkable man faced the difficulty
and overcame it. He was not by training a
philologist or scholar ; but he made himself one.
And so we see him in his other phase, as the

industrious student engaged in the dull, hard, endless grind which alone could equip the language of the Old Testament for use in the present-day book and newspaper, in the home and street, in the theatre and public meeting. A huge Hebrew literature, from the Song of Deborah to the poems of Bialik, had to be dredged and sifted for forgotten words which could meet modern requirements ; roots must be dug out from Hebrew and the cognate languages, and be refashioned and refurnished as derivatives to give the most concrete of ancient tongues an elasticity that could cope with the abstractness of so much of to-day's thought ; yet, again, new words had to be created to name the new ideas and the new material of modern life.

"An Idea Achieved.

" This work went on hand in hand with Ben Yehudah's public propaganda : almost every day in his newspapers and conversation he introduced new words, new turns of phrase, which contributed to the vitality and possibilities of the language. At an early stage in his career he saw the pressing need of a dictionary which should embody all the vocabulary of Hebrew of every age and his own (and others') innovations. He made several tentative efforts, from small vocabularies in the columns of his earliest newspaper to a dictionary of moderate scale. Finally, he planned a Thesaurus on a plan scarcely less grandiose in scale than the great Oxford English Dictionary. This he had nearly completed by the time of his death. The fifth volume of the *Thesaurus totius hebraitatis et veteris et recentioris* was published in 1921 ; five further volumes were planned, together with two introductory volumes describing the historical evolution of the language, and these, it is understood, were left in a condition requiring little further labour to render them fit for publication. This work is now being done.

" Eliezer ben Yehudah's life is a rare example of a life's ideal achieved. During the first 20 years he spent in Palestine he was looked upon as crazy. The most famous of his contemporaries poured scorn on his queer idea of reviving so mouldered a corpse. Only 15 or 20 years ago spoken Hebrew was still a thing of scorn and derision in Palestine. It was mere ' Ben Yehudah language ', the whim of a madman. When Ben Yehudah tried to address Lilienblum, then the greatest apostle of Jewish revival, in Hebrew, he was met by the contemptuous snub, *Redet wie a Mensch,* Yiddish for ' Talk like a reasonable being '. But he lived to see the world of his dream ; he lived to see newspapers attacking him for his political heresies, yet in every sentence and paragraph using words, phrases, and terms of abuse of his own creating ; he lived to see the new Jerusalem, with its entertainments, theatrical performances, operas, public speeches, scientific discussions—all in spoken Hebrew. He lived to see Hebrew recognized as an official language of the Government of his ' home ' country, the official publication in Hebrew of a Parliamentary ' White Paper ', the insertion of a clause in the terms of the British Mandate over Palestine protecting the rights of Hebrew, and a census return according to which 96 per cent. of the Jews of Palestine declared Hebrew to be their mother-tongue."

CHAPTER IX

THE WILL AS A DETERMINANT

WITHOUT the will, or with the will so weak as to be ineffective, the individual is a mere automaton, irresponsible, ungoverned—a ship drifting with wind and tide. The pleasure principle may furnish the chief determinant which will co-operate with or be opposed by other determinants, some of which are unknown to the individual being hidden in the unconscious mind. That these hidden determinants may be of great potency Freud has shown, though we dissent from his view that determinism reigns supreme. But it is true that without the exercise of the will a man drifts at the mercy of determinants. To express the matter truly we must include the will as one of the determinants. This, of course, assumes the psychic energy which the will directs. In using the expressions, a " *strong* will " or a " *weak* will " we are intending to connote the available energy behind the will in a particular case.

Having indicated how futile is the argument by which Freud attempts to show that our consciousness of free-will is a delusion, we proceed on the supposition that the will is just as real a component of the motivation of actions as are the other components. We use the word components advisedly because the determinants are additive, some plus and some minus, and it is the sum which determines the resulting action. The will brings in a determinant, plus or minus, which goes into the total.

It is quite true, as Freud tells us, that the motivation of action is often obscure, but whilst Freud would lead us to imagine that we had no control over these determinants we shall show later how the will can not only act directly but also indirectly by enabling us to build up determinants for ourselves.

The motives which determine action are often very complex. Some lie quite open to our consciousness in the upper stratum of the mind. We recognize conflicting motives there. For instance we see that duty may lie in one direction and inclination in another. We are conscious of this conflict of motives which is open and above board. The will may be weak and we may consciously put aside duty and act upon inclination. Or the will may be sufficiently powerful to enable us to follow duty in spite of inclination. But in addition to the conscious motives which puzzle the will there are the unconscious and unrecognized motives which are often the strongest, the seat of which is the unconscious mind. The conflicting motives whose interplay takes place in the field of consciousness may be likened to two opposing counsel pleading in open court before the judge who has to decide and act. But motives hidden in the unconscious mind impart a powerful bias to the judge of which he is unconscious. Their voice is not heard in open court. The bias is unrecognized and therefore all the more potent. Where the will is weak and the unconscious bias is strong the bias takes charge and determines the decision. It may, according to its nature, either reinforce the weak will to right and determine a right decision or it may overpower the weak will and determine a wrong decision. The opposing counsel pleading in the open court of consciousness are up against a hidden factor which is both unrecognized and unsuspected. The judge does not decide the case merely upon the force of their pleadings but under the influence of a bias hidden in the unconscious mind which may make either for a right or wrong decision.

For the sake of clearness we may formulate some of the propositions involved :—

    1. Action at a given crisis is the resultant of several determinants, viz., the will, the conflicting motives which are weighed in

the forum of consciousness and the unconscious motives arising from the unconscious mind.

2. The will may be so severely handicapped by unconscious motives as to be entirely over-borne by them, or, on the other hand, it may be so reinforced by them as to turn the scale in the right direction when the critical moment for action arrives.

3. Everything which is fixed in the unconscious mind tends to influence judgment, decision, or action independently of the will.

4. Thoughts, ideas and mental pictures which are voluntarily entertained with approval sink into the unconscious mind and become springs of action or determinants.

It will simplify matters if we regard not only the will but all the other motives and unconscious determinants as deflectors of energy. They are so many hands grasping the rudder lines of the human boat. Some pull one rope and some the other, and the angle which the rudder takes and the consequent course which is steered depend upon the combined effect of the various forces.

Now this metaphor will help us to make clear an important point in reference to the most efficient use of the will. If you are steering a boat in a race and have to get round a bend in the course, you do not wait till you are opposite to the bend and then put on a lot of rudder sharply. If you do you will very likely run into the opposite bank, and in any case you will take a lot of way off the boat. You put on as little rudder as is necessary and keep it on steadily so as to take you in a smooth curve round the bend. Now with a strong will it may be possible to make an energetic use of it when the moment for action arrives, but with risks, and in the case of a weak will, with the certainty of disaster if the opposing determinants are strong. But even a weak will can be steadily and continuously used *in anticipation of the emergency*, to build up determinants which will reinforce the will and enable you to keep the desired course when the occasion arises with a minimum of will effort at the moment. It is no doubt true that a weak will is at the mercy of opposing determinants. What the Freudian theory fails to grasp is that, whilst we may be more or less at the mercy of determinants at the decisive moment, *we ourselves can mould those determinants*. No one can afford to rely solely upon the sudden directive agency of the will coming into action unexpectedly along with a number of other determinants unknown and of unknown strength. But a prolonged application even of a comparatively weak will can create determinants which will be effective where a sudden application of the will power available at the moment might be unavailing.

In the next chapter we shall indicate the way in which definite auto-suggestion may be used to secure this result. Here we may point out that unconscious suggestion is an important element in the formation of determinants, but even over unconscious suggestion our attitude of approval or disapproval gives us control.

Everyone is more or less motivated by the ideal which he sets before himself. This ideal is largely the creation of

> Education
> Books
> Lectures
> Conversation
> Friendships and
> Environment generally.

From all these things come suggestions which if *approved and appropriated*, act auto-suggestively, build up ideals and form determinants in the unconscious which will operate in due course. We shall deal later with active auto-suggestion which is consciously used. We speak here of external suggestions which we approve *ambulando* and unconsciously appropriate. This belongs largely to the domain of education, which is dealt with by other writers, but the point to be made is that it is a factor in *self-education* and should be thoroughly understood and borne in mind for our own guidance, unless we wish to be at the mercy of determinants thoughtlessly created.

To avoid books, conversation, friendships and environments which are detrimental to the ideal which we keep before us, requires a comparatively small but persistent exercise of will-power. To choose books, friends and an environment generally which is favourable to the growth of our ideal again requires only a small application of will-power. But the constant directive exercise of the will for these purposes will make all the difference to the determinants which we acquire and which will operate in conjunction with or against the will when occasion arises.

Many people drift at the mercy of their environment, without exercising any definite choice in the matter of friendships, books, etc. These things are more or less left to chance or to the determination merely of the pleasure principle. It is not realized that the sum of all these things creates important and permanent determinants which will either help or hinder progress towards the ideal which in thoughtful moments they cherish. Of course, many people do not take enough interest in themselves and what they are becoming to trouble about what they

are becoming—what individuality they are daily
building up. The pursuit of pleasure, of sport,
of money, takes off their attention from themselves, and the final result in themselves. But
for those who keep before themselves some ideal
towards which they wish to grow, the importance
of the determinants which are being unconsciously built up day by day should not be
overlooked.

Such determinants are also produced from
day to day in the course of the smaller conflicts
and struggles of daily life. If the directive
force of the will is continuously used in the right
way, determinants are stored up in the power-
house of the unconscious with a directive effort
of will which is almost unconscious when the goal
is kept steadily in view. And so for the emer-
gencies of life, the will should be chiefly used in
continuous generation of determinants—habits
of mind, thought and action—which will operate
automatically when the occasion arises without
making much call on the will at the moment.
In fact, one may say that for the average man
one of the chief uses of the will is in the slow and
patient creation of determinants day by day.

CHAPTER X

By auto-suggestion powerful determinants may be planted in the unconscious mind with a minimum of demand upon the will, which determinants may be of great use in helping the will when the maximum demand is made upon it. We have already spoken of external or environmental suggestion which operates almost unconsciously. It is probable that external suggestion is only operative when it is so far approved and appropriated as to become auto-suggestion. But this requires little if any effort of the will. When a boy reads the story of Dick Turpin, if his critical faculty is so far dormant that he approves and admires, the suggestion may operate to prompt him to like deeds. But we are now concerned with definite auto-suggestion which may be consciously used for various purposes. Such suggestion may, in the first place, be external, but if it be adopted it becomes auto-suggestion without making any great call upon the will.

Thus, suppose a schoolmaster desires to

illustrate the effect of suggestion to the boys in a dormitory and suggests to them by way of experiment that in the morning at an untimely hour he will give three knocks on the door, upon which without waiting to think about it every boy is to jump quickly out of bed. It may be found that with half the boys it operates and with the others not. For those who adopted the suggestion and assimilated it, it will act auto-suggestively. For the rest the response may be feeble.

A suggestion may often be effective where a resolution would fail. We may take an illustration of this from the personal experience of the writer, who was accustomed for some years to go by train to London and then take a walk of something less than a mile to the Temple. The walk was performed automatically in an unvaried way, attention during the walk being given to the work of the day and entirely abstracted from perambulation. Now under these circumstances a resolution formed over night to depart from the beaten track in order to make an exceptional call on the way was usually forgotten. The Temple would be reached automatically and the slip of memory not realised until then. It was found that such a slip could be obviated by the following procedure. When the intention was formed the point at which divergence from the beaten track became necessary was forcefully pictured in the imagination—a street corner or a crossing or some other point on the beaten track which could not be missed. Then the mental suggestion was made—" When you reach that point, you are to pause and think—what next ? You are to diverge from the beaten track and pursue another course (also forcefully pictured in the imagination) until you arrive at the desired objective ". If this auto-suggestion was carried out sufficiently carefully it had the desired effect, *without any further effort*. The suggestion would disappear from consciousness, but when next day the point of divergence was reached, the suggestion would at once spring into consciousness and be carried out.

This is merely an illustration from the writer's own experience of how a sufficiently powerful auto-suggestion sinks into the unconscious and is motivated from the unconscious by the postulated stimulus. Here the amount of will-power required was very small. All that was wanted was a clear intention, and a clear-cut mental picture of the way in which it was to be carried out. No strain upon the will was involved. The suggestion took the form of a series of commands, automatically obeyed when the time came.

The carrying out of a resolution involves often

a considerable effort of the will both in the making and to perform it when the time comes. But a suggestion in the form of a command to oneself, which may be repeated and emphasized to be sure that it sinks in, requires comparatively little effort of the will either in the making or in the carrying of it out. Moreover the psychic effect of a resolution broken is damaging, whereas the effect of a suggestion not followed is much less serious and the suggestion can be repeated till it is carried out.

One may illustrate the *modus operandi* further by two other experiences. The writer wished to try the effect of an *unspoken* suggestion upon a hypnotised person. The suggestion was that he should walk to the other end of the room, pick out a particular hat from a dozen or more lying on a table and put the hat on his head. The *modus operandi* was to stand a little way behind the hypnotized subject and to think forcibly, which meant saying internally with mental emphasis but without speech : " You are to go forward. Go further forward. Put out your hand. A little more to the right. Pick up the hat below your hand. Put it on your head ". These unspoken commands were obeyed. Here we have the suggestor and the actor separated into two distinct persons. The suggestive command passed through the unconscious mind of the actor and was carried out *without any effort of will on* his part—thus illustrating how a determinant implanted by suggestion in the unconscious mind requires no will-power to carry it out. Get the suggestion fixed there and it will operate. Moreover the suggestion involves very little will-power on the part of the suggestor. To give a command to yourself or to anybody else need not involve any strain of the will. It only involves definiteness and precision of thought.

Another experiment was made on a subject in a normal state, but who was specially receptive to telepathic impressions. The suggestion made was to walk to the middle of the room, reach up to a tap in a chandelier over-head and turn off the gas. The unspoken commands were somewhat as follows : " Go forward, a little to the left, stop, lift up your hand, a little higher, more to the right, grasp the tap there, turn it ". These commands were obeyed. In this case as in the preceding case there was no contact and no other indication given than by thought. The command of the suggestor was obeyed by the actor, without any strain of the will in giving the command and with no effort of will on the part of the actor. All he did was (as he expressed it) to " keep his mind a blank " and obey any impressions which came into it.

There is little doubt that in cases of telepathy the impression is received by the unconscious mind and that any thoughts of the conscious mind tend to interfere with it.[1]

These cases illustrate how a suggestion planted in the unconscious mind becomes a determinant which operates without any exercise of the will of the actor.

Freud tells us that he has found both hypnotic suggestion and ordinary suggestion of little use in his psycho-therapeutic treatment, though he agrees that the phenomenon of " transference " between the patient and physician may act to some extent by suggestion. But it would seem that there must be cases in which direct suggestion may be of marked utility under certain conditions.

The condition that the suggestion should be turned into auto-suggestion, appears to be vital. If the patient can be induced to adopt the suggestion and repeatedly re-suggest it to himself it may be of high efficacy. If the patient is really anxious to be cured and is made to understand how auto-suggestion plants determinants in the unconscious which will, as it were, do their own fighting when they are fixed there, he will be

---

[1] A fuller account of these experiments is to be found in an article by the writer on telepathy in the *Hibbert Journal*, April, 1922.

ready to do his best to co-operate. For instance suggestion may be used, *with the co-operation of the patient*, as a help in overcoming a vicious habit which may form part of a pathogenic complex. Its value is that it does not depend *on good resolutions*. The making of *a resolution* to do something unpleasant or abstain from doing something pleasurable raises a counter-effect of doubt in the mind which may deprive the resolution of its force. But an auto-suggestion in the form of a command to one's self: " You will do so and so " or " You will not do so and so ", or other appropriate suggestion suited to the case, even if it fail once or twice, may succeed in the end if the patient is really in earnest in repeating the suggestion time after time. The first failures will be put down to the auto-suggestion, the self-command, not having been sufficiently forcible and the effect of a broken resolution will be avoided. If it fails in one form ingenuity will suggest another form in which it may succeed, but all of course depends on exciting the patient's interest in the matter. He will also gain confidence if he practises simple auto-suggestions having nothing to do with his neurosis and easily carried out which will show him the *modus operandi* of the method.

Again it should be noted that there are many

things which may act suggestively in opposition
to the influence of the physician against which
the patient should be warned. A patient who is
troubled with excess of erotic energy, in reading
erotic literature easily adopts in imagination the
rôle of the objectionable character—lives the
part in imagination—and so sets up a mischievous auto-suggestion which creates or enhances
erotic energy. A warning from the physician is
surely desirable in such cases. Also the patient
should be shown the importance of controlling
his own thoughts, and imaginings, and should
be made to understand that active thinking in
the wrong direction will hinder his progress.
Where the patient suffers from excess of erotic
energy, which has been suppressed, he should be
made to understand clearly that when he suffers
his imagination to play around erotically he is
turning psychic energy into the erotic channel
and so creating the excess from which he suffers.
And the resources of psychology can give
practical directions to the patient for shutting off
this hurtful imaginative activity.

Furthermore there are many cases in which
the patient has a morbid or hopeless or materialistic outlook upon life. In such cases one can
hardly expect the materialist to make suggestions which will give a hopeful outlook which
envisages a life beyond. But the judicious

psycho-analyst who is not a materialist will
often be able to give suggestions which will
brighten the patient's outlook on life and give
him a wider horizon.	Failing this the patient
who has had brought to light things of which
he never dreamed may be so oppressed by the
disclosures that the last state of the patient may
be worse than the first.

No doubt the making of suggestions on the
religious side is a delicate and difficult thing,
best left alone unless the psycho-analyst himself
has a fundamentally religious outlook on life.
Anything in the nature of dogma would be quite
out of place.	But the religious ideas embodied
in the parables of the Prodigal Son and the Good
Samaritan, for instance, are such as would give
many patients the new outlook on life which
they require.	Dr. R. M. Riggall, a well-known
psycho-analyst says : "Used in conjunction
with psycho-analysis physicians find that religion
is a great help in dealing with the neuroses".
And Dr. Paul Bousfield "recognises that all
forms of religion are for many patients valuable
channels of sublimation".	This, of course, is
quite contrary to Freud's teaching, according
to which, after having laid bare the conflict and
the repressions, "The conditions of symptom
formation are abolished and the pathogenic
conflict exchanged for a normal one which must

be decided one way or another. Nothing is done for the patient except to make this one mental change take place in him.

" The analyst refrains from playing the part of mentor. He wants the patient to find his own solutions for himself ".

All this ignores the fact that in the conflict between erotic energy and its antagonist a new outlook on life may be of the first importance.

A quotation from the Translator's preface to Jung's *Psychological Types* (p. ix) will further indicate the wide difference from Freud's view which exists among psycho-analysts.

" It has been argued that psycho-analysis does not claim to be more than a therapeutic technique and a method of research, and that it is irrelevant for the psychologist to concern himself with the question of human development or with the inevitable ancillary problems of morality, religion and human relationship. In this very argument the essential limitations of this standpoint stand self confessed, since a psychology that excludes the most vital problems of life from its sphere of responsibility requires no further criticism. It is already moribund. Actually, of course, a psychological nihilism which broke down every individual form into its elements and put nothing in its place could not conceivably have anything but disastrous therapeutic results. But Freud does put something definite and positive in its place, for there always remains the transference to the analyst which, in the case of a positive transference, involves a gradual assimilation by the patient to the analyst's general attitude to life, and in the alternative case a very definite rejection of the man and all his ways. This unconscious identification with the analyst is quite outside the sphere of the latter's control. It is inherent in the analytical relationship. But for the analyst to wash his hands of this unconscious effect, is as irresponsible as though a surgeon were to shut his eyes to the inevitable dangers of hæmorrhage and sepsis. The question of moral responsibility is therefore inherent in analytical practice ".

Perhaps it is as well that materialistic psycho-analysts should limit themselves as Freud does to laying bare the causes of the neurosis. The oulook on life of the materialist is the last thing that should be assimilated by the patient. Let us welcome the birth of a new generation of psycho-analysts who will not suffer from the compulsion ideas of the materialistic complex.

CHAPTER XI

CONCLUSIONS

IT will be convenient to summarize some of the chief conclusions at which we have arrived in the course of our criticism of the Freudian psychology.

The Materialistic Complex with its compulsion ideas is a pathological condition which is the result of a conflict in which the idea of moral responsibility becomes painful and is repressed. Associated ideas, such as those of free will, God, or a future existence, are also drawn into the complex. Hence arise compulsion ideas which are the negations of these associated ideas.

The Materialistic Complex, like other complexes, disables the intellect from functioning normally in relation to any matters which touch the complex. The sufferer refuses to entertain opinions or ideas in conflict with the compulsion ideas of the complex. Evidence which runs counter to the complex is rejected, or neglected, or trifling excuses are made for putting it on one side. For conclusions in conformity with the complex very slight evidence suffices. Specious analogies which support the compulsion ideas are seized upon without perception of their insufficiency. The sufferer is in complete ignorance of the complex, although his arguments, decisions and opinions in matters which it touches are entirely moulded by it, and at the same time his intellectual capacity in other matters may be of a high order.

Freud's treatment of the subjects of free will and "superstitions" shows all the symptoms of the materialistic complex, which dictates the conclusions at which he arrives, and leads him to put forward what are mere personal opinions as deductions which are scientifically demonstrated.

In his *Psycho-pathology of Every-day Life* he cites a number of cases in which actions are motivated from the unconscious. In all these cases there is involved no effort of the will. Yet he draws the inference that free-will is a delusion from the analogy of cases in which the will is not a factor.

Cases in which the will does in fact overcome opposing determinants are ignored by Freud, yet such incidents are facts of experience. Freud regards this experience as illusive, upon no other ground than the analogy of cases in which the will is inoperative.

Freud has shown in *Totem and Taboo*, that

elementary ideas of spirit, survival, morality and unseen powers existed among primitive races in all parts of the world. These ideas have evolved with the evolution of the race and are still held by the majority of mankind. *Prima facie* these ideas correspond to realities and the burden of proof that they are illusions is upon those who say so. According to Freud these ideas are comparable with the compulsion ideas of neurotics. But he shows no justification for interpreting normal human minds, whether primitive or civilized by the mentality of neurotics. To regard the normal as a phase of the abnormal is unscientific. The analogy with neurotics breaks down when Freud attempts to apply it.

Freud regards the psyche as a function of the soma and the highest qualities in man as derivatives of the sexual instincts. This theory breaks down when it is applied to *amor*—the love that "seeketh not its own" and is purely philanthropic. There is no justification for regarding this as a somatic derivative. This break-down of the theory can only be patched up by regarding the philanthropic type (including the Christ-type) as neurotic, a view for which there is no psychological justification.

Freud regards psychic energy as a derivative of sexual energy, and aims at the sublimation of sexual energy and its diversion into non-sexual channels. He fails to point out that erotic energy is generated by the play of the imagination upon sexual matters, and he gives no warning against this. He fails to perceive that by this play of the imagination upon sexual matters psychic energy is diverted into lower channels. He therefore fails to grasp that the true aim should be not merely the sublimation of erotic energy, but the prevention of its creation.

Freud's post-analytical treatment aims at health, but character is a secondary consideration. If character alone survives, it should be a primary consideration. "A psychology which excludes the most vital problems of life from its sphere of responsibility requires no further criticism". There are many cases in which post-analytical suggestions would be valuable, such, for instance, as would open a new outlook on life or teach the patient how to avoid the generation of erotic energy. But if the analyst has a materialistic outlook the patient will assimilate this to his undoing, in which case it may be well for the analyst to leave the patient to "find his own solutions".

We have used the term psyche to denote that which survives when the soma disintegrates. For our purpose it was not necessary to consider it as soul and spirit on theological lines. Character includes the attributes of the psyche which survive. If man were not the master of his actions, if these were solely the result of determinants implanted by heredity and environment, a man would have no responsibility for his character. Nations also would be irresponsible since the character of a nation is the integration of the characters of its members.

The growth of character depends upon the results of the conflicts of everyday life. These are not sham fights in which the will is powerless. There are, of course, many cases in which the will is overcome by determinants, but the will must be reckoned as one of the determinants. Action is the resultant of all the conflicting determinants, conscious and unconscious, including the will. The will can control the formation of determinants in the unconscious which may operate in its aid.

Freud has taught us to look at the unconscious mind as a power-house which gives out the strongest determinants of conduct. He has failed to point out that the contents of this power-house, when a person has reached the age at which serious conflicts begin, are largely under his own control.

The fact that sexual restrictions and the notion of survival appear in the very dawn of humanity is of the highest significance. The conflicts which arise out of the sexual instincts are the strongest and the mode in which these are met chiefly determines character. These instincts can be controlled by control of the imagination. The repression of erotic imaginings is not a pathogenic repression, and will prevent the generation of erotic energy which might involve pathogenic repression. The sexual instincts which in the animal stage of evolution served a reproductive purpose now serve the higher purpose of a field of conflict in which the highest character may be developed.